Cellular and Molecular Aspects of Fiber Carcinogenesis

SERIES EDITORS
John Inglis and Jan A. Witkowski
Cold Spring Harbor Laboratory

CURRENT COMMUNICATIONS
In Cell & Molecular Biology

CURRENT COMMUNICATIONS

2

In Cell & Molecular Biology

Cellular and Molecular Aspects of Fiber Carcinogenesis

Edited by

Curtis C. Harris
National Cancer Institute

John F. Lechner
National Cancer Institute

B.R. Brinkley
University of Alabama
at Birmingham

 Cold Spring Harbor Laboratory Press 1991

CURRENT COMMUNICATIONS 2
In Cell & Molecular Biology
Cellular and Molecular Aspects of Fiber Carcinogenesis

Front Cover: Differential interference-contrast photomicrograph of two living pneumocytes from the newt *Tarlcha granulosa* that were cultured for 65 hours in the presence of crocidolite asbestos fibers. The large size, flat morphology, and optically clear cytoplasm make newt pneumocytes highly suited for examining the incorporation and subsequent behavior of asbestos within the living cell. In this example, both pneumocytes contain numerous fibers that ultimately become concentrated around the cell nucleus. (Courtesy of C.L. Rieder. See related article by Rieder et al., this volume.)

Back cover: Rat pleural mesothelial cells in culture treated with 1 µg/cm^2 of chrysotile fibers for 48 hours. Numerous fibers are seen in the cell. (Courtesy of M.C. Jaurand and L. Kheuang, INSERM U139, Créteil).

Library of Congress Cataloging-in-Publication Data

Cellular and molecular aspects of fiber carcinogenesis / edited by
    Curtis C. Harris, John F. Lechner, B.R. Brinkley.
        p. cm. — (Current communications in cell and molecular
    biology ; 2)
        Includes index.
        ISBN 0-87969-361-4
        1. Lungs—Cancer—Etiology. 2. Mesothelioma—Etiology.
    3. Inorganic fibers—Carcinogenicity. 4. Mesothelioma—Molecular
    aspects. 5. Asbestosis—Molecular aspects.   I. Harris, Curtis C.,
    1943 - .   II. Lechner, John F.   III. Brinkley, B. R.   IV. Series.
    RC280.L8C43   1991
    616.99'424071--dc20   91-9478
                                                                               CIP

The articles published in this book have not been peer-reviewed. They express their authors' views, which are not necessarily endorsed by Cold Spring Harbor Laboratory.

All Cold Spring Harbor Laboratory Press publications may be ordered directly from Cold Spring Harbor Laboratory Press, 10 Skyline Drive, Plainview, New York 11803. Phone: 1-800-843-4388. In New York (516) 349-1930. FAX: (516) 349-1946.

Contents

Preface

The adverse health effects of airborne fibers are a major environmental concern. Naturally occurring mineral fibers such as asbestos are well-known occupational hazards, but whether or not substitute fibers, including man-made substances, also present risks is uncertain. A major theme of this volume is the pathobiological comparison of asbestos with other types of fibers, including its proposed substitutes.

Fiber toxicity has been strongly implicated in carcinogenesis of the lungs, yet many questions about the association remain unanswered. There is uncertainty in extrapolating pathobiological effects from a high to a low fiber dose, due in part to the small size of the data base compared with those from studies of chemical carcinogens or radiation. The physical dimensions and stability of asbestos may also be important in the pathogenesis of bronchogenic carcinoma, mesothelioma, and asbestosis, with implications for the potential hazards of substitute fibers. Oxy-radicals and growth factors are released by macrophages activated by fibers in various lung diseases, and the cytoskeleton and mitotic spindle apparatus are physically disrupted by long and thin fibers; the importance of these events in cytotoxicity and carcinogenesis is unclear. It is not known whether the synergy between high exposure to asbestos and tobacco smoke found in occupational settings operates in people exposed to lesser amounts of asbestos or substitute fibers. In addition, the molecular basis for the abnormally high oncogenic and cytotoxic susceptibility of mesothelial cells is unexplained.

To answer these questions, including those related to risk assessment, a multidisciplinary effort is required. There is a special need for increased understanding of the molecular mechanisms of fiber-induced aberrations in cell division, transduction of growth factor signals, and genomic stability. The status of these fundamental studies is another major theme of this book.

Background chapters are provided by Rom, Knuutila (see Tiainen et al.), and Hesterberg et al. Rom shows that asbestos induces the release of bioresponse modifiers and speculates on their possible role in asbestos-caused disease. Knuutila demonstrates that patterns are emerging among the complex karyotypes of mesothelioma cells. Monosomy of chromosomes 22, 1, 3, and 9, polysomy of chromosomes 7 and 11, and structural abnormalities of chromosomes 1, 3, and 7 are relatively common in mesotheliomas, and the greater the number of chromosomes 7, the worse the prognosis. Hesterberg describes preliminary data from inhalation studies of man-made mineral fibers showing that some fibers are detectably carcinogenic in Syrian hamsters, but not in rats.

Other chapters deal with growth factors, signal transduction and the cytoskeleton, and the design of studies on the effect of fibers on these mechanisms. Molloy et al. discuss the current understanding of mitogenesis induced by platelet-derived growth factor (PDGF), which has been incriminated in mesothelioma. Brody considers the biological activity of a group of polypeptide hormone-like cytokines that have been collectively called growth factors, particularly the factors synthesized and secreted by lung macrophages exposed to fibers. Rheinwald (see O'Connell and Rheinwald) reports that human mesothelial cells incubated in the presence of epidermal growth factor (EGF) produce interleukin-1 and colony-stimulating factors. In addition, he presents evidence that mutant Ha-*ras*-transformed human mesothelial cells no longer require EGF for replication.

Mitotic spindle control and aberrations are described by Rieder, Sluder, and Brinkley (see Rieder et al.). These authors review current concepts of mitosis and chromosome movement and identify possible routes of asbestos-induced aneuploidy. Brinkley presents recent investigations on the organization of centrioles, the kinetochore, and centromeres, and Sluder contributes recent data on centrosomes and shows that centrioles can replicate without a nucleus. Sluder also suggests that the presence of a fiber within the mitotic spindle probably affects the timing of mitosis. Rieder describes how kinetochore malfunction can lead to aneuploidy and speculates that centrioles might attach to fibers, forming a pseudo-aster that captures chromosomes and prevents their migration to the metaphase plate. Finally, Barrett shows that mutant p53 leads to Syrian hamster embryo (SHE) cells with indefinite population-doubling potentials. In addition, he notes that aneuploidy (commonly a gain in chromosome 11) tightly correlates with transformation of SHE cells. The DNA of mesothelioma cells has transforming activity in 3T3 cells, but the gene(s) responsible has not been identified.

Mossman and Marsh contribute a chapter on molecular mechanisms. They find that animals exposed to asbestos after receiving catalase minipump implants have fewer macrophages in their lung lavage fluid, less hydroxyproline synthesis in their lungs, and less severe pathology than control animals. The data implicate the iron component of the fibers in these asbestos effects, suggesting that ferruginous bodies may not be as innocuous as thought previously. Jurand et al. report that cultured rat pleural epithelial cells can be transformed with asbestos, but the emergence of tumorigenic cells requires many population doublings. Hei et al. report a strong synergism between asbestos and X-rays in causing transformation of 10T1/2 cells and also describe experiments showing that asbestos alone is mutagenic via a clastogenic mechanism. Lechner et al. report that the growth of human mesothelial cells in general can be stimulated by numerous peptide antigens but that there appears to be considerable inter-individual variation in responsiveness to the mitogens. They also describe the "immortalization" of a nontumorigenic human mesothelial cell line, MeT-5A, that can be transformed to tumorigenicity by transfection with mutant Ha-*ras* but not by amosite asbestos. Furthermore, Lechner et al. show that human mesotheliomas express both PDGF A-chain or PDGF B-chain mRNAs, whereas normal cells express only the A-chain. In addition, preliminary observations with MeT-5A cells suggest that cells transfected with A-chain vector constructs over-expressed A-chain mRNA and are tumorigenic, whereas cells given the B-chain vector remain nontumorigenic. These authors also describe amosite-induced spindle integrity infidelity in human mesothelial cells. Finally, Walker et al. report that cultured rat mesothelial cells do not express transforming growth factor-α, PDGF A-chain, or PDGF B-chain mRNAs.

Mesothelioma cells show similar gene expression, but insulin receptor mRNA is not expressed. Walker et al. also note that cultured mesothelioma cells readily acquire polysomy of chromosome 1.

Before preparing their contributions to this volume, the authors had the benefit of a stimulating discussion meeting on the theme at the Banbury Conference Center of Cold Spring Harbor Laboratory. The success of the meeting was enhanced by the scientific and administrative efforts of Jan Witkowski and Bea Toliver of the Banbury Center, the gracious hospitality of Katya Davey, hostess of Robertson House, and the many corporate sponsors who supported it financially. The expertise of John Inglis, Nancy Ford, Ralph Battey, Inez Sialiano, and their co-workers at Cold Spring Harbor Laboratory Press was essential for the timely publication of this volume.

C.C.H.
J.F.L.
B.R.B.

Special Support

The meeting at the Banbury Center on which this book is based was supported by funding from:

Environmental Protection Agency
Thermal Insulation Manufacturers Association (TIMA)
ILSI Risk Science Institute (RSI)

Corporate Sponsors

The meetings' program at Cold Spring Harbor Laboratory is supported by:

Alafi Capital Company
American Cyanamid Company
AMGen Inc.
Applied Biosystems, Inc.
Becton Dickinson and Company
Boehringer Mannheim Corporation
Bristol-Meyers Squibb Company
Ciba-Geigy Corporation/Ciba-Geigy Limited
Diagnostic Products Corporation
E.I. du Pont de Nemours & Company
Eastman Kodak Company
Genentech, Inc.
Genetics Institute
Hoffmann-La Roche Inc.
Johnson & Johnson
Kyowa Hakko Kogyo Co., Ltd.
Life Technologies, Inc.
Eli Lilly and Company
Millipore Corporation
Monsanto Company
Pall Corporation
Perkin-Elmer Cetus Instruments
Pfizer Inc.
Pharmacia Inc.
Schering-Plough Corporation
SmithKline Beecham Pharmaceuticals
The Wellcome Research Laboratories,
    Burroughs Wellcome Co.
Wyeth-Ayerst Research

Some Possible Routes for Asbestos-induced Aneuploidy during Mitosis in Vertebrate Cells

C.L. Rieder,[1,2] **G. Sluder,**[3] **and B.R. Brinkley**[4]

[1]Wadsworth Center for Labs and Research, New York State
Department of Health, Albany, New York 12201
[2]School of Public Health, State University of New York
Albany, New York 12222
[3]Worcester Foundation for Experimental Biology, Shrewsbury
Massachusetts 01545
[4]Department of Cell Biology and Anatomy, University of Alabama at
Birmingham, Alabama 35294

INTRODUCTION

Asbestos and other mineral fibers have long been implicated in the etiology of various diseases including lung cancer and mesotheliomas of the pleura, pericardium, and peritoneum (Wagner et al. 1974; Stanton et al. 1981; for review, see Mossman et al. 1990). However, despite much research, the mechanism(s) by which these fibers promote oncogenesis remain obscure (Craighead 1987; Barrett et al. 1989). Unlike most carcinogens, asbestos does not appear to be mutagenic (Weisburger and Williams 1981; Casey 1983; Oshimura et al. 1984; Kenne et al. 1986). It may, however, act as a tumor promoter in the presence of other suspected carcinogens (Topping and Nettesheim 1980; Mossman et al. 1983). Alternatively, since asbestos treatment by itself produces bronchogenic carcinomas and mesotheliomas (Wagner et al. 1974; Stanton et al. 1981), and since fiber dimensions appear as important as composition in transforming cells (Stanton et al. 1981; Hesterberg and Barrett 1984; for review, see Mossman et al. 1990), asbestos may affect cells by more direct mechanisms. In this respect, aneuploidy is such a common characteristic of

Cellular and Molecular Aspects of Fiber Carcinogenesis
Copyright 1991 Cold Spring Harbor Laboratory Press 0-87969-361-4/91 $1.00 + 00

asbestos-induced tumors that it has been hypothesized that such a shift in chromosome complement plays a major role in the early stages of immortilization and neoplastic progression (Lechner et al. 1985; Oshimura et al. 1986; Libbus and Craighead 1988; for review, see Oshimura and Barrett 1986; Barrett et al. 1990).

Aneuploidy is commonly defined as a lack (hypoploidy) or excess (hyperploidy) of individual chromosomes (Sybenga 1972). As detailed by Oshimura and Barrett (1986; see also Liang and Brinkley 1985), this condition can be produced by numerous agents, most of which are chemicals whose targets include, e.g., DNA replication, chromosome condensation and paring, and components of the cytoskeleton and spindle apparatus. However, asbestos is relatively inert, and once inside the interphase cell, it appears to be accumulated preferentially in the perinuclear region (Fig. 1A) (Barrett et al. 1989). As a re-

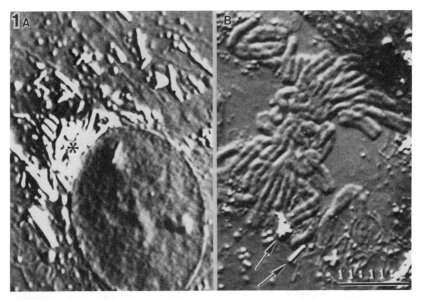

FIGURE 1 Selected micrographs from time-lapse, differential-interference-contrast video light microscopy sequences of living newt (*Taricha granulosa*) pneumocytes cultured in the presence of crocidolite asbestos. (A) An interphase cell in which the incorporated birefringent asbestos fibers are concentrated primarily in the perinuclear region (asterisk). (B) A prometaphase cell that contains two asbestos fibers (arrowheads) in the vicinity of the forming spindle. Bar, (B) 25 μm.

sult, it is not uncommon to find asbestos fibers within or near the mitotic apparatus of dividing cells (Fig. 1B) (Jaurand et al. 1983; Hesterberg and Barrett 1985; Kenne et al. 1986; Wang et al. 1987; Barrett et al. 1989). These observations and the fact that dimensions are more important than composition in the transforming potency of the fibers have led to the hypothesis that asbestos induces aneuploidy primarily by interfering with the normal course of mitosis (Oshimura et al. 1984; Hesterberg and Barrett 1985; Hesterberg et al. 1986; Kenne et al. 1986; Palekar et al. 1987; Wang et al. 1987; Barrett et al. 1989). Our purpose here is to summarize our current concepts of how the spindle forms and functions in vertebrate cells and then to outline some possible mechanisms by which asbestos may disrupt chromosome distribution during mitosis.

MITOTIC SPINDLE OF VERTEBRATE CELLS

The mitotic spindle of vertebrate cells consists of an ensemble of structures whose principles are diagramed in Figure 2. The two ends or "poles" of the normally bipolar spindle contain centrosomes that nucleate radial arrays of microtubules (MTs) known as asters. These astral arrays serve to anchor the spindle in the cytoplasm. Spindle formation in vertebrate somatic cells results from an interaction between the spindle poles and specialized structures on each chromatid that are known as kinetochores (for review, see Rieder 1990). As a result of this interaction, bundles of MTs are constructed that firmly connect the two chromatids of a replicated chromosome to opposite spindle poles. In addition to these kinetochore fiber (K-fiber) MTs, the spindle also contains numerous non-K-fiber MTs that are derived from the overlapping arrays of astral MTs (a thorough discussion of spindle structure can be found in McDonald [1989]).

Spindle Poles

Since the structure, function, and composition of centrosomes have been reviewed recently (Wheatley 1982; Vandre and Bori-

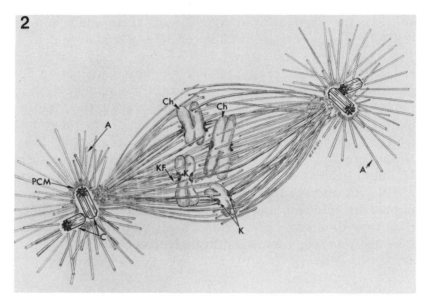

FIGURE 2 Schematic diagram of a vertebrate metaphase spindle showing the principal structural components of the mitotic apparatus. (C) Centrioles; (PCM) pericentriolar material; (K) sister kinetochores; (Ch) chromosomes; (KF) kinetochore fiber microtubules; (A) astral microtubules. See text for details.

sy 1989; Rieder 1990; Sluder 1990a), this topic is only briefly summarized here. With few exceptions, the centrosome of vertebrate cells consists of a pair of centrioles (i.e., a diplosome), the oldest of which is typically associated with a primary cilium and a prominent cloud of fibrogranular pericentriolar material (PCM) containing numerous, densely staining pericentriolar satellites (Fig. 3A,B). During interphase, the PCM nucleates the assembly of numerous cytoplasmic MTs. Most but not all of these MTs coexist in growing and shrinking populations (i.e., they exhibit dynamically unstable behavior; Mitchison and Kirschner 1984; Cassimeris et al. 1988). In cycling cells, the centrosome is replicated near the time of DNA synthesis in preparation for the impending mitosis. Throughout the remainder of interphase, the replicated centrosomes usually remained linked (Fig. 3A,B) and behave as a single

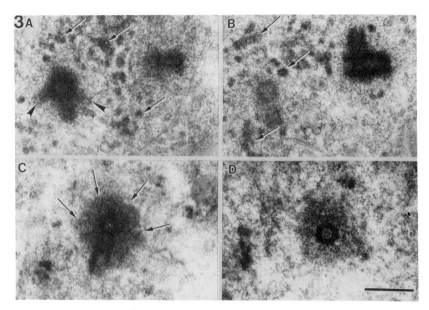

FIGURE 3 High-voltage electron micrographs of serial 0.25-μm-thick sections through the centrosome of a late interphase (*A,B*) and a mitotic (*C,D*) PtK cell. The replicating late-interphase centrosome contains two pairs of centrioles in close proximity. The oldest centriole of this centrosome possesses centriolar appendages (*A*, arrowheads) and is surrounded by pericentriolar material and satellites (*A,B* arrows). By contrast, the metaphase centrosome (*C,D*) possesses a more extensive cloud of pericentriolar material (*C*, arrows) and fewer satellites. To better visualize centrosomal structures, the microtubules associated with both of these centrosomes were disassembled prior to fixation by a cold shock. See text for details. Bar, (*D*) 0.5 μm. (Reprinted, with permission, from Rieder and Borisy 1982.)

unit. As the cell enters mitosis, the cytoplasmic MTs and many of the ancillary structures associated with the replicated centrosomes are resorbed concomitantly with the phosphorylation of some centrosomal proteins and an expansion of the PCM surrounding the diplosome (Fig. 3C,D) (for review, see Rieder 1990). These structural and chemical changes correlate with a functional change in that each of the replicated centrosomes now generates a radial "astral" array of MTs. When compared with the interphase centrosome, the astral arrays of dynamically unstable MTs generated by the mitotic centrosomes contain substantially more but shorter MTs (Vandre and Borisy 1989).

Kinetochore

The kinetochore is responsible for attaching the chromosome to the forming spindle and is actively involved in generating the forces for chromosome motion (Gorbsky et al. 1987; Nicklas 1989; Rieder and Alexander 1990). In view of their essential role in chromosome movement, kinetochores are likely targets for aneuploidogenic compounds (Brinkley et al. 1985). Since kinetochore composition, structure, and function have been reviewed recently (Mitchison 1988; Brinkley et al. 1989; Pluta et al. 1990; Sluder 1990b), only those aspects that currently appear relevant to spindle formation and chromosome motion will be summarized here.

Each replicated chromosome contains a single pair of (sister) kinetochores, one of which is associated with each chromatid (Fig. 4). As a rule, these kinetochores are positioned on opposite sides of the replicated chromosome and are separated from one another by the width of the primary constriction. The structure of the vertebrate "disk" kinetochore varies depending on whether it is associated with and attached to the spindle by K-fiber MTs. Unattached kinetochores appear as moderately electron-opaque rectangular or circular plate-like structures (Fig. 4A), approximately 40–60-nm thick, that vary widely in diameter depending on the species (e.g., see Brinkley et al. 1984). This plate is composed of numerous, tightly interwoven chromatin filaments and associated proteins. In all cases, a conspicuous fibrous "corona" is associated with and radiates a variable distance from the surface of the kinetochore plate (Fig. 4A) (for review, see Brinkley et al. 1989; Rieder 1990). The kinetochore is separated from but firmly connected to the underlying heterochromatin of the primary constriction by an electron-translucent region traversed by a low density of chromatin fibrils. The availability of human autoantibodies directed against the centromere/kinetochore region (Fig. 4B) (Moroi et al. 1980) has enabled investigators to identify and characterize some of the functional proteins associated with

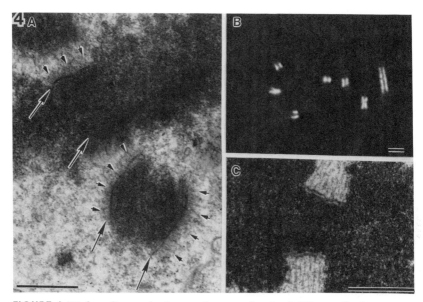

FIGURE 4 High-voltage electron micrograph of a 0.25-μm-thick section through the primary constriction of several PtK chromosomes from a cell arrested in mitosis with colcemid. This section was treated with 10 nm of colloidal gold fudiciary particles. The sister kinetochores (arrows) appear as plate-like structures on opposite sides of the primary constriction. Note the fibrous corona material (arrowheads) that radiates a variable distance from each plate. (*B*) Indirect immunofluorescence micrograph of an Indian muntjac chromosome complement (2*N* = 7) stained with human antisera directed against the kinetochore/centromere complex. Note that the length of the kinetochore complexes vary widely between chromosomes. (*C*) Electron micrograph of a thin section through the sister kinetochore region of an Indian muntjac metaphase chromosome. Many of the kinetochore fiber microtubules terminate on the outer plate of the kinetochore, which lacks the fibrous corona material. See text for details. Bars: (*A*) 1.0 μm, (*B*) 1.0 μm, (*C*) 1.0 μm.

this structure (Balczon and Brinkley 1987; for review, see Brinkley et al. 1989; Brinkley 1990; Pluta et al. 1990).

Kinetochores undergo two obvious structural changes as K-fiber MTs associate with and terminate within or on the kinetochore plate (Fig. 4C) (for review, see Rieder 1990). First, the kinetochore becomes significantly reduced in size. Second, the corona material appears greatly diminished or nonexistent. However, if those K-fiber MTs terminating on the kinetochore (i.e., kinetochore MTs) are disassembled by various (chemical or physical) treatments, the size of the kinetochore plate increases and the fibrous corona once again becomes a conspicuous feature of the kinetochore (Cassimeris et al. 1990).

Spindle Formation and Function

Spindle bipolarity, which is crucial for ensuring that the chromatids are equally distributed, is established by the separation of replicated centrosomes. The mechanism(s) responsible for this separation are unknown, but the event itself may occur prior to, during, or well after nuclear envelope breakdown (NEB) (for review, see Rieder and Hard 1990). Regardless of when the centrosomes separate, the initial behavior of a chromosome at NEB is, as a rule, predicted by its position relative to the spindle pole(s). If centrosome separation fails completely or if it is delayed until well after NEB, all of the chromosomes form a monopolar attachment and move into the single polar region. In contrast, if centrosome separation is initiated prior to or during NEB, those chromosomes positioned approximately halfway between them at NEB frequently acquire a rapid bipolar connection. Under these conditions, chromosomes positioned significantly closer to one spindle pole at NEB generally first attach and then move toward that pole prior to achieving a bipolar attachment and congressing toward the forming metaphase plate (Fig. 5). Regardless of the route by which the spindle forms, the temporal order of chromosome attachment is dictated by proximity to a pole, i.e., those chromosomes closer to a pole at NEB attach well be-

FIGURE 5 (*A–H*) Selected frames from a time-lapse differential-interference-contrast video light microscopy sequence of a newt (*T. granulosa*) pneumocyte undergoing mitosis. After nuclear envelope breakdown (*A–B*), many of the chromosomes monoorient to the closest pole (*C*, arrows). Over time, all but one of these chromosomes form a bipolar attachment and congress to the metaphase plate (*D–F*). In this cell, one monooriented chromosome (*F–H*, arrows) fails to initiate congression prior to the onset anaphase (*G–H*) and as a result, both the daughter cells produced by the division are aneuploid. Time is at lower right hand corner of each micrograph. Bar, (*H*) 25 μm.

fore those more distally located (for review, see Rieder 1982). In this respect, the attachment of a chromosome well removed from the closest spindle pole at NEB may be delayed for

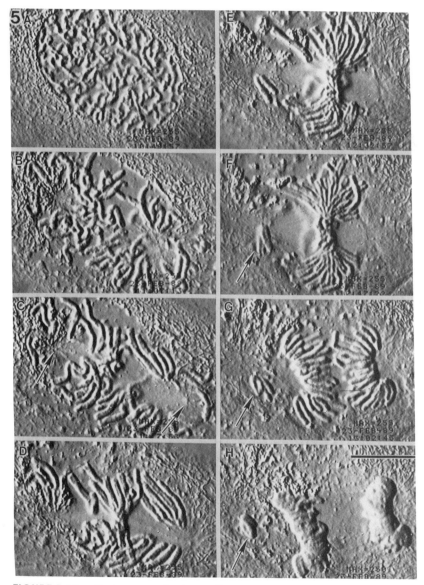

FIGURE 5 (*See facing page for legend.*)

several hours, or it may even fail to attach (Rieder and Alexander 1990).

Recent work has directly demonstrated that chromosome attachment occurs when one of the kinetochores on the chromosome interacts with the surface of or end of a single astral MT (Hayden et al. 1990; see also Rieder and Alexander 1990). As a consequence of this interaction, the now monooriented chromosome is transported toward the astral center (i.e., into a region of progressively higher MT density) where additional MTs are rapidly incorporated into the forming K-fiber. In cases where the chromosome attaches well away from the polar area, it may become detached from the spindle during poleward transit (due to the lability of the initial MT-kinetochore interaction; Alexander and Rieder 1991). As a rule, however, these chromosomes rapidly reattach and complete their poleward journey. These findings imply that all of the MTs used to construct the vertebrate mitotic spindle are ultimately derived from the asters (Hayden et al. 1990).

The initial monopolar attachment and the resulting rapid (up to 60 μm/min; Alexander and Rieder 1991) movement of the chromosome into the closest spindle pole is a prevalent feature of prometaphase in vertebrate cells. This monoorientation event occurs in response to the formation of a K-fiber on only one kinetochore of the chromosome. Recent immunological evidence (Pfarr et al. 1990; Steuer et al. 1990) supports the hypothesis that this movement is mediated by cytoplasmic dynein bound to corona fibrils that extend from the surface of the kinetochore plate (Rieder and Alexander 1990). In turn, these dynein "motor" molecules work against kinetochore-associated MTs to move the chromosome pole-ward. Current thinking favors the idea that dynein provides the force responsible for both the rapid movements of attaching chromosomes along the surface of astral MTs and the slower congression and anaphase movements when the kinetochores are attached to the ends of one or more MTs.

To be equally distributed during the ensuing anaphase, monooriented chromosomes must ultimately acquire an attachment to the distal pole and undergo congression movements to the equator of the forming spindle (Fig. 5). It has been argued (e.g., Rieder 1990) that this process is facilitated by the continual growth of densely packed astral MTs within the spindle, which tend to "push" associated chromosomes away from the centrosome and toward the metaphase plate. As a consequence of this "astral ejection force," the monooriented chromosome will, at some point in prometaphase, become positioned closer to the distal pole, where it is much more likely to encounter MTs growing from that pole.

Once a chromosome acquires a bipolar attachment, it undergoes complex congression movements as the opposing K-fibers on the sister kinetochores mature. This maturation of K-fibers correlates with a diminution of chromosome velocity (i.e., fully formed K-fibers of prometaphase and anaphase cells move chromosomes >25x slower than nascent K-fibers; Alexander and Rieder 1991), and culminates in the metaphase alignment of the chromosome. The manner in which spindle forces on opposite daughter chromatids are balanced to bring a chromosome to the center of the spindle is not fully understood. For meiotic cells, Hays and co-workers (Hays et al. 1982; Hays and Salmon 1990) present evidence consistent with a length-tension model in which the poleward force on a kinetochore is a function of the number and length of kinetochore-associated MTs. This model requires that kinetochore-associated MTs act as traction fibers having force-producing elements along their length and that these MTs disassemble at the spindle poles. However, recent data from spermatocytes and somatic cells reveal that the poleward force generated in association with kinetochore MTs is produced primarily at the kinetochore (Gorbsky et al. 1987; Nicklas 1989; Rieder and Alexander 1990) and that these MTs disassemble or shorten at the kinetochore (Mitchison et al. 1986; Gorbsky et al. 1987; Nicklas 1989). Thus, the equilibrium position of chromosomes on the spindle equator cannot be simply a function of MT number and length. Indeed, the centering of a bipolar-oriented chromosome at the metaphase plate appears to result from a combination of independent forces including equal pulling forces generated by daughter kinetochores and aster ejection forces, acting along the length of the chromosome, that are balanced midway between the poles of the spindle (Carlson 1938; Rieder et al. 1986; Salmon 1989b,c).

Regardless of the mechanism by which the forces are produced and balanced, the congression movements of a chromosome to the metaphase plate requires that the K-fiber MTs attached to one kinetochore elongate, whereas those attached to the other (sister) kinetochore coordinately shorten. Similarly, K-fiber MTs must shorten when an anaphase kinetochore moves toward a pole during anaphase. Recent microinjection (Mitchison et al. 1986), fluorescence recovery after photobleaching (Gorbsky et al. 1987), and micromanipulation (Nicklas 1989) experiments reveal that the length changes of kinetochore MTs, in response to prometaphase and anaphase chromosome movements, occur primarily by the addition and deletion of MT subunits at the kinetochore. The rate at which the kinetochores remove or add tubulin subunits may "govern" chromosome velocity (for review, see Nicklas 1983; Rieder and Alexander 1990). How tubulin subunits enter and exit MT ends that are mechanically anchored in the kinetochore is an intriguing problem for future investigation (see, e.g., Mitchison 1988).

In general, cells containing even a single, monooriented chromosome spend an inordinate amount of time in prometaphase waiting for it to congress (Zirkle 1970a). In these cases, the cell apparently "senses" that a chromosome has yet to achieve a proper orientation and delays the onset of anaphase. Preliminary data of Zirkle (1970b) suggest that the control function for this delay resides in the unattached kinetochores and is not due to the absence of the kinetochore from the metaphase plate. However, the cell cannot wait an indefinite period of time to conclude its division, as evidenced by the fact that it will ultimately enter anaphase even in the presence of one or more maloriented chromosomes (Fig. 5) (Rieder et al. 1986). Thus, entry into anaphase is partly governed by a timing mechanism or a sequence of events that are sensitive to but cannot be overridden by a maloriented chromosome (see, e.g., Rieder and Alexander 1989). In this context, potorous tridactylus kidney (PtK) cells normally complete their mitosis within 1–2 hours; however, they remain in mitosis for up to 8 hours in the presence of agents (e.g., colcemid and nocodazole) that disrupt MT assembly (the role of spindle MTs in the timing of mitotic events is discussed in Sluder 1979, 1988; Sluder and Begg 1983).

The initiation of anaphase is signaled by the disjunction of sister chromatids. This disjunction process is not due to an increase in poleward forces on the chromatids, since chromosome splitting occurs in the complete absence of spindle MTs (Mole-Bajer 1958; Mazia 1961; Sluder 1979). Recent work on chromosomal proteins that appear to hold sister chromatids together prior to anaphase was discussed in Cooke et al. (1987) and Earnshaw and Cooke (1989). Once disjoined, the anaphase chromatids begin to move slowly (~2 μm/min) toward the poles to which they are attached (anaphase A). During this time, the distance between the spindle poles is also increased (anaphase B). The force-producing mechanism for anaphase A remains to be elucidated, but it is likely based on the same (cytoplasmic dynein) motors responsible for the poleward movement of monoorienting prometaphase chromosomes. The mechanism for spindle elongation during anaphase B is similarly unknown. It may result from a push generated by the sliding of interacting and interdigitating MTs of opposite polarity, arising from the opposing asters (as in the diatom spindle; see, e.g., Cande et al. 1989), or it may be the result of a pull generated independently by each aster as its MTs interact with the cell cortex (see, e.g., Bajer 1982).

In late anaphase or early telophase, the cell begins to cleave. The cleavage apparatus consists of a circumferential band of actin filaments that interacts with cytoplasmic myosin to contract much like a drawstring. The position of the cleavage furrow on the cell cortex is determined by the two asters at the time of anaphase onset in ways that are not well understood (for review, see Rappaport 1986; Salmon 1989a). Once initiated, cleavage is usually complete within 30 minutes, although the newly formed daughter cells may remain connected for several hours by a narrow cytoplasmic channel known as the stem body.

SOME POSSIBLE ROUTES FOR FIBER-INDUCED ANEUPLOIDY DURING MITOSIS

General Considerations

For the most part, mineral fibers are thought to be incorporated into cells by phagocytosis (Suzuki et al. 1972; Suzuki

1974), during which time they are encased in a portion of the plasma membrane. As a result, at the electron microscopy level it is common to see such fibers surrounded by membrane (Fig. 6) (Jaurand et al. 1983) or within phagosomes (Jaurand et al. 1983), and even forming asbestos bodies may be surrounded by membrane (see, e.g., Suzuki 1974). However, in other cases asbestos fibers appear to lack an associated membrane (e.g., Fig. 6). Whether all or only some asbestos fibers are demembranated once inside the cell, the mechanism and time course of this process, and whether this process is dependent on the size and/or type of asbestos and/or cell are currently unknown and are important considerations for ultimately understanding the mechanism(s) by which asbestos affects the mitotic process.

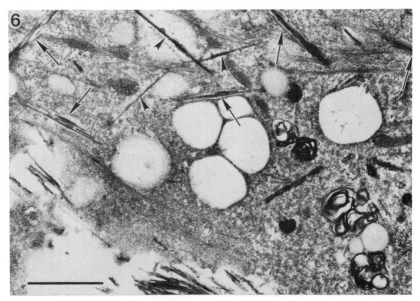

FIGURE 6 Electron micrograph of a thin section through the cytoplasm of a newt (*T. granulosa*) pneumocyte that has incorporated Calidria chrysotile asbestos fibers. Many of the fibers are surrounded by membranes (arrows), whereas some are not (arrowheads). Bar, 2.0 μm.

Asbestos fibers less than 1 μm in diameter and more than 4 μm long appear most effective at inducing neoplasms in vivo and in vitro (Stanton et al. 1981; Hesterberg and Barrett 1984; for review, see Mossman et al. 1990). This size dependency may reflect factors such as the ability of fibers to reach cells deep within the lung, the selective loss of the phagocytic membrane surrounding larger fibers, and the fibers having a sufficient size to perturb the mitotic process effectively.

The primary karyotypic change associated with asbestos-induced carcinomas appears to be the loss or gain of one (Oshimura et al. 1986) or a few chromosomes (Oshimura et al. 1984, 1986; Lechner et al. 1985; Craighead et al. 1987; Libbus and Craighead 1988). The conclusion that the oncogenetic properties of asbestos or glass fibers are not related to their composition, but size (see Introduction and above) strongly supports the contention that these insoluble mineral fibers do not interfere with spindle function by chemically "poisoning" one or more key processes such as chromosome condensation, chromatid disjunction, MT formation, and so forth. Indeed, cultured cells can undergo multiple rounds of normal divisions in the presence of asbestos fibers (Keene et al. 1986). Thus, one of the likely ways in which asbestos fibers induce aneuploidy is by mechanically interfering with the normal course of mitosis in a small proportion of cells, and the gain or loss of chromosomes then leads to the transformation of those cells that have genetic changes compatible with growth (see references in Introduction). The asbestos fibers that are responsible for the original chromosomal shift may then be progressively "diluted" (Kenne et al. 1986) during subsequent divisions to the point where the aneuploid cells no longer contain asbestos.

Once within the cell, mineral fibers do not appear to be incorporated into the interphase or prophase nucleus. As a result, their physical effects on mitosis must be restricted to the time between NEB and nuclear envelope reformation in late anaphase. In addition, their effects on mitosis should be most evident in cells whose spindles are most susceptible to interference from cytoplasmic inclusions. In this respect, mesothelial cells appear much more sensitive to asbestos than other types of epithelia (for discussion, see Mossman et al.

1983; Lechner et al. 1985). In culture, rapidly dividing meso-thelia lack keratin filaments (Connell and Rheinwaldi 1983), whereas other types of epithelia often contain a cage of keratin filaments surrounding the interphase and mitotic nucleus (Mandeville and Rieder 1990). In some cases, this keratin cage can be clearly demonstrated to act as a barrier to prevent cyto-plasmic organelles (and perhaps asbestos) from invading the forming spindle.

There are at least two distinctly different physical properties of asbestos fibers that may confer aneuploidy-producing capa-bilities through mechanical means. These include steric con-siderations related to fiber size, and the ability of the fiber to interact with cytoplasmic components through charge-charge interactions. These two properties may work independently or synergistically to effect chromosome distribution.

Steric Considerations

The spindle is a very dynamic structure that undergoes rapid rocking and rotational movements within the cytoplasm as it forms (for review, see Rieder and Hard 1990). During this time, chromosomes may also be moving toward or away from a pole. Thus, the spatial relationships between asbestos fibers, within the cytoplasm and spindle, and the chromosomes are in con-stant change throughout the mitotic process. Once within the spindle, asbestos fibers may inhibit the normal process of chromosome segregration, at any stage, by sterically blocking normal chromosome attachment or disrupting normal motion (Hesterberg and Barrett 1985; Palekar et al. 1987; Wang et al. 1987).

When positioned at NEB between a spindle pole and one or more chromosomes, the larger fibers could generate aneuploi-dy by prohibiting astral MTs from contacting the kinetochores or by "holding" a chromosome out of the range of the forming spindle. As a result, the duplicated chromosome would be left stranded in the cytoplasm during anaphase. Even if such a chromosome became attached to the spindle, it could become permanently detached as it moves poleward by impacting a fiber, or it could be similarly prevented from forming a bipolar connection and congressing. Although possible, such a "shielding" mechanism would predict that increasing the fiber diameter would enhance their capacity to induce aneuploidy, which is a prediction that is not supported by the observation that thin fibers are much more aneuploidogenic than thicker ones (see above). However, even small fibers that are especially long could immobilize "lost" chromosomes that are ejected well distal to the region of the forming spindle during NEB and prevent them from wandering (via cytoplasmic currents) into the casting range of the aster.

The tendency of the forming spindle to expel large objects toward its periphery is thought to be mediated by the dynamically unstable behavior of astral MTs (Rieder et al. 1986; Salmon 1989b). However, thin, linear asbestos fibers that achieve an orientation parallel to spindle MTs should not be eliminated, but instead should become permanently trapped within the forming spindle. Under these conditions, such fibers would be well positioned to contact attaching or congressing chromosomes. On forceful contact, the fiber may penetrate or pierce the chromosome which in turn may then adhere strongly (in the absence of a membrane) to the fiber because of mutual charge interactions or fiber-surface irregularities. As a result, the kinetochore or K-fiber might be severed or damaged, or the forces generated by the spindle (which are on the order of 10^{-6} dyn; Nicklas 1983; Alexander and Rieder 1991) may be insufficient to overcome the additional drag imparted on the chromosome by the fiber. Either event could disrupt (1) the subsequent bipolar attachment of a monooriented chromosome, (2) the congression movements and final equilibrium position of a bipolar, attached chromosome, and/or (3) the normal disjunction and poleward movement of anaphase chromosomes (to produce laggards and chromatin bridges). Each of these routes could ultimately lead to chromosome breakage or aneuploidy, and all of these are consistent with published studies of cells dividing in the presence of asbestos (e.g., see Fig. 1 of Hesterberg and Barrett 1965; Fig. 4 of Palekar et al. 1987).

Alternatively, long fibers, which penetrate the spindle perpendicular to its long axis, may be ultimately locked into place by cytoskeletal components (e.g., keratin) surrounding the forming spindle. Under these conditions, the asbestos could physically block poleward chromosome motion by bisecting K-fibers or chromosomes.

In addition to disrupting normal chromosome motion sterically, asbestos fibers no doubt mechanically inhibit the completion of cleavage when positioned between the separating groups of anaphase chromosomes. In this regard, cytoplasmic inclusions that are external to the metaphase spindle are often seen to "flow" into the midzone as chromosomes complete their anaphase movements and the cell begins to cleave (Rieder and Hard 1990). Once in this location, asbestos fibers would produce tetraploid or binucleated cells by acting as a physical barrier to the completion of cytokinesis. This scenario is strongly supported by the preponderance of binucleated polyploid cells after exposure to asbestos in vitro (Jaurand et al. 1983; Kenne et al. 1986; Palekar et al. 1987).

Charge-Charge Interactions

The surface of some asbestos fibers (e.g., chrysotile) is positively charged and shows a high affinity for polar proteins (for review, see Mossman et al. 1983; Wang et al. 1987). It is therefore possible that some of the key soluble proteins involved in mitosis adhere to asbestos. For example, fibers may become coated with tubulin and MT-associated proteins to provide an MT-mimicking surface along which the kinetochores of chromosomes can move, as suggested by the ability of glass pipettes to substitute for MT bundles in supporting bidirectional organelle movement in *Echinosphaerium* (Edds 1975). If a kinetochore moves along a mineral fiber that is not directed toward the spindle, the chromosome may move into the cytoplasm and never attach to the spindle. Similarly, such fibers may have a high preferential affinity for certain key proteins involved in chromosome attachment and out-compete other spindle components for such proteins. Because of their charge properties, demembranated asbestos fibers may also stick tenaciously to various structural components of the spindle (e.g., see Jaurand et al. 1983; Oshimura et al. 1984; Hesterberg and Barrett 1985). When attached to MTs or chromatin they may disrupt normal chromosome segregation as outlined above. Alternatively, the PCM responsible for nucleating the MTs that form the spindle may stick to demembranated asbestos during interphase as the centrosomes are replicated. Under these circumstances, each fiber may act as an ancillary spindle pole to which one or more chromosomes attach and subsequently move.

Although such charge-charge interaction hypotheses are attractive, they are admittedly quite speculative and are complicated by a lack of general information. For example, since asbestos fibers are usually incorporated into interphase cells, they should be coated first with interphase proteins (which may or may not be essential to mitosis). Can those proteins unique to and essential for mitosis replace interphase proteins, absorbed on the fiber, that are not involved in mitosis? Similarly, any interaction between fibers and chromosomes or spindle components that is based on such an absorption scheme is difficult to imagine if the fiber is encased in a phagocytic membrane. As previously noted, the fate of the phagocytic membrane surrounding incorporated asbestos is currently unknown.

Timing of Mitotic Events

In addition to disrupting mitosis by steric hindrance or their charged properties, asbestos fibers may have more subtle but equally devastating effects on the timing of mitotic events. Spindle MTs are not only necessary for the execution of most mitotic events, but also play a key role in the mechanisms that control the timing of these processes. If spindle MTs are rearranged (Sluder and Begg 1983) or are prevented from assembling (Sluder 1979; for review, see Sluder 1988), the mitosis phase of the cell cycle is greatly prolonged or arrested. If MT assembly is diminished, mitosis proceeds significantly slower than normal. Therefore, if mineral fibers transiently disturb the ionic balance of the cell, e.g., by punching holes in the plasmalemma when the cell is moved during breathing, spindle assembly could be prevented or diminished. Such an event during mitosis may lead to malorientation or nondisjunction of individual chromosomes. Importantly, prolongation of mitosis results in the splitting of unreplicated centrosomes before the completion of mitosis (Sluder 1979; Keryer et al. 1984; Sluder and Begg 1985) to produce tripolar or tetrapolar spindles that have obvious consequences for chromosome distribution.

SUMMARY

It is well established that mineral fibers can interfere with the segregation of chromosomes during mitosis. However, the mechanisms by which these fibers perturb this process remain to be elucidated. Given the complexity of the mitotic process and the many points at which mineral fibers can interfere, we feel that it would be naive to expect that fiber-induced aneuploidy (and consequently cell transformation) is produced by only a single mechanism. We freely admit that many of the possibilities we outline are speculative, but all are plausible. As cell biologists and microscopists, we perceive an important need to examine further these issues systematically and completely, using newly developed light and electron microscopy methodologies currently employed by the students of mitosis. Past attempts to examine the behavior of asbestos fibers in individual living cells undergoing mitosis, which could directly evaluate these hypotheses, have not proven successful. This appears primarily because of the fact that the cells chosen for analyses (CHO, Kenne et al. 1986; rat pleural mesothelial cells, Jaurand et al. 1983) have small diameter and round considerably during cell division, obscuring the relationships between the fibers and the mitotic apparatus. Similar studies, using newly developed, video-enhanced light microscopy methods (for review, see Inoue 1986) and larger lung cells, which remain flat throughout mitosis (see, e.g., newt pneumocytes; Rieder and Hard 1990; Fig. 1), may provide important data relevant to these questions. We are excited by the possibility that an interdisciplinary effort will generate a clearer understanding of the ways in which mineral fibers effect chromosome distribution during mitosis.

ACKNOWLEDGMENTS

The authors thank Mr. R. Cole for his assistance with the asbestos studies on newt lung cells, Mr. A. DeMarco for his darkroom assistance, Mr. F.J. Miller for his artwork, and Dr. T.M. Fasy for providing us with asbestos fibers. This work was supported in part by National Institutes of Health (NIH) grant GM-40198 to C.L.R., GM-30758 to G.S., CA-41424 to B.R.B., and NIH grant PHS-01219, which was awarded by the Department of Health and Human Services/Public Health Service, to support the Wadsworth Center's Biological Microscopy and Image Reconstruction Facility as a National Biotechnological Resource.

REFERENCES

Alexander, S.P. and C.L. Rieder. 1991. Chromosome motion during attachment to the vertebrate spindle: The initial saltatory-like behavior of chromosomes and a quantitative analysis of nascent kinetochore fiber force production. *J. Cell Biol.* (in press).

Bajer, A.S. 1982. Functional autonomy of monopolar spindle and evidence for oscillatory movement in mitosis. *J. Cell Biol.* **93:** 33.

Balczon, R.D. and B.R. Brinkley. 1987. Tubulin interaction with kinetochore proteins: Analysis by in-vitro assembly and chemical crosslinking. *J. Cell Biol.* **105:** 855.

Barrett, J.C., P.W. Lamb, and R.W. Wiseman. 1989. Multiple mechanisms for the carcinogenic effects of asbestos and other mineral fibers. *Environ. Health Perspect.* **81:** 81.

Barrett, J.C., D.G. Thomassen, and T.W. Hesterberg. 1990. Role of gene and chromosomal mutations in cell transformation. *Ann. N.Y. Acad. Sci.* **407:** 291.

Brinkley, B.R. 1990. Centromeres and kinetochores: Integrated domains on eukaryotic chromosomes. *Curr. Opin. Cell Biol.* **2:** 446.

Brinkley, B.R., A. Tousson, and M.M. Valdivia. 1985. The kinetochore of mammalian chromosomes: Structure and function in normal mitosis and aneuploidy. In *Aneuploidy* (ed. V. Dellarco et al.) p. 243. Plenum Press, New York.

Brinkley, B.R., M.M. Valdivia, A. Tousson, and R.D. Balczon. 1989. The kinetochore: Structure and molecular organization. In *Mitosis: Molecules and mechanisms* (ed. J.S. Hyams and B.R. Brinkley), p. 77. Academic Press, New York.

Brinkley, B.R. M.M. Valdivia, A. Tousson, and S.L. Brenner. 1984. Compound kinetochores of the Indian muntjac: Evolution by linear fusion of unit kinetochores. *Chromosoma* **91:** 1.

Cande, W.Z., T. Baskin, C. Hogan, K.L. McDonald, H. Masuda, and L. Wordeman. 1989. In vitro analysis of anaphase spindle elongation. In *Cell movement: Kinesin, dynein and microtubule dynamics* (ed.

F.D. Warner and J.R. McIntosh), vol. 2, p. 441. A.R. Liss, New York.

Carlson, J.G. 1938. Mitotic behavior of induced chromosomal fragments lacking spindle attachments in the neuroblasts of the grasshopper. *Proc. Natl. Acad. Sci.* **24:** 500.

Casey, G. 1983. Sister-chromatid exchange and cell kinetics in CHO-K1 cells, human fibroblasts and lymphoblastoid cells exposed in vitro to asbestos and glass fibre. *Mutat. Res.* **116:** 369.

Cassimeris, L., N.K. Pryer, and E.D. Salmon. 1988. Real time observations of microtubule dynamic instability in living cells. *J. Cell Biol.* **107:** 2223.

Cassimeris, L., C.L. Rieder, G. Rupp, and E.D. Salmon. 1990. Stability of microtubule attachment to metaphase kinetochores in PtK$_1$ cells. *J. Cell Sci.* **96:** 9.

Connell, N.D. and J.G. Rheinwaldi. 1983. Regulation of the cytoskeleton in mesothelial cells: Reversible loss of keratin and increase in vimentin during rapid growth in culture. *Cell* **34:** 245.

Cooke, C.A., M.M.S. Heck, and W.C. Earnshaw. 1987. The inner centromere protein (INCENP) antigens: Movement from inner centromere to midbody during mitosis. *J. Cell Biol.* **105:** 2053.

Craighead, J.E. 1987. Current pathogenetic concepts of diffuse malignant mesothelioma. *Human Pathol.* **18:** 544.

Craighead, J.E., N.J. Akley, L.B. Gould, and B.L. Libbus. 1987. Characteristics of tumors and tumor cells from experimental asbestos-induced mesothelioma in rats. *Am. J. Pathol.* **129:** 448.

Earnshaw, W.M. and C. Cooke. 1989. Proteins of the inner and outer centromere of mitotic chromosomes. *Genome* **31:** 541.

Edds, K.T. 1975. Motility in *Echinosphaerium necleofilum*. 1. An analysis of particle motions in the axopodia and a direct test of the involvement of the axoneme. *J. Cell Biol.* **66:** 145.

Gorbsky, G.J., P.J. Sammak, and G.G. Borisy. 1987. Chromosomes move poleward in anaphase along stationary microtubules that coordinately disassemble from their kinetochore ends. *J. Cell Biol.* **104:** 9.

Hayden, J., S.S. Bowser, and C.L. Rieder. 1990. Kinetochores capture astral microtubules during chromosome attachment to the mitotic spindle: Direct visualization in live newt lung cells. *J. Cell Biol.* **111:** 1039.

Hays, T.S. and E.D. Salmon. 1990. Poleward force at the kinetochore in metaphase depends on the number of kinetochore microtubules. *J. Cell Biol.* **110:** 391.

Hays, T.S., D. Wise, and E.D. Salmon. 1982. Traction force on a kinetochore at metaphase acts as a linear function of kinetochore fiber length. *J. Cell Biol.* **93:** 374.

Hesterberg, T.W. and J.C. Barrett. 1984. Dependence of asbestos- and mineral dust-induced transformation of mammalian cells in culture on fiber dimension. *Cancer Res.* **44:** 2170.

————. 1985. Induction by asbestos fibers of anaphase abnormalities: Mechanism for aneuploidy induction and possibly carcinogenesis. *Carcinogenesis* **6**: 473.

Hesterberg, T.W., C.J. Butterick, M. Oshimura, A.R. Rody, and J.C. Barrett. 1986. Role of phagocytosis in Syrian hamster cell transformation and cytogenetic effects induced by asbestos and short and long glass fibers. *Cancer Res.* **46**: 5795.

Inoue, S. 1986. *Videomicroscopy.* Plenum Press, New York.

Jaurand, M.C., I. Bastie-Sigeac, J. Bignon, and P. Stoebner. 1983. Effect of chrysotile and crocidolite on the morphology and growth of rat pleural mesothelial cells. *Environ. Res.* **30**: 225.

Kenne, K., S. Ljungquist, and N.R. Ringertz. 1986. Effects of asbestos fibers on cell division, cell survival, and formation of thioguanine-resistant mutants in Chinese hamster ovary cells. *Environ. Res.* **39**: 448.

Keryer, G., H. Ris, and G.G. Borisy. 1984. Centriole distribution during tripolar mitosis in Chinese hamster ovary cells. *J. Cell Biol.* **98**: 2222.

Lechner, J.F., T. Tokiwa, M. LaVeck, W.F. Benedict, S. Banks-Schlegel, H. Yeager, A. Banerjee, and C.C. Harris. 1985. Asbestos-associated chromosomal changes in human mesothelial cells. *Proc. Natl. Acad. Sci.* **82**: 3884.

Liang, J.C. and B.R. Brinkley. 1985. Chemical probes and possible targets for the induction of aneuploidy. In *Aneuploidy* (ed. V. Dellarco et al.), p. 491. Plenum Press, New York.

Libbus, B.L. and J.E. Craighead. 1988. Chromosomal translocations with specific breakpoints in asbestos-induced rat mesotheliomas. *Cancer Res.* **48**: 6455.

Mazia, D. 1961. Mitosis and the physiology of cell division. In *The cell: Biochemistry, physiology, morphology* (ed. J. Brachet and A.E. Mirsky), p. 77. Academic Press, New York.

Mandeville, E.C. and C.L. Rieder. 1990. Keratin filaments restrict organelle migration into the forming spindle of newt pneumocytes. *Cell Motil. Cytoskel.* **15**: 111.

McDonald, K. 1989. Mitotic spindle ultrastructure and design. In *Mitosis: Molecules and mechanisms* (ed. J. Hyams and B.R. Brinkley), p. 1. Academic Press, New York.

Mitchison, T.J. 1988. Microtubule dynamics and kinetochore function in mitosis. *Annu. Rev. Cell Biol.* **4**: 527.

Mitchison, T. and M. Kirschner. 1984. Dynamic instability of microtubule growth. *Nature* **312**: 237.

Mitchison, T., L. Evans, E. Schulze, and M. Kirschner. 1986. Sites of microtubule assembly and disassembly in the mitotic spindle. *Cell* **45**: 515.

Mole-Bajer, J. 1958. Cine-micrographic analysis of c-mitosis in endosperm. *Chromosoma* **9**: 332.

Moroi, Y., C. Peeples, M.J. Fritzler, J. Steigerwald, and E.M. Tan.

1980. Autoantibody to centromere (kinetochore) in scleroderma sera. *Proc. Natl. Acad. Sci.* **77:** 1627.

Mossman, B.T., W.G. Light, and E.T. Wei. 1983. Asbestos: Mechanisms of toxicity and carcinogenicity in the respiratory tract. *Annu. Rev. Pharmacol. Toxicol.* **23:** 595.

Mossman, B.T., J. Bignon, M. Corn, A. Seaton, and J.B.L. Gee. 1990. Asbestos: Scientific developments and implications for public policy. *Science* **247:** 294.

Nicklas, R.B. 1983. Measurements of the force produced by the mitotic spindle in anaphase. *J. Cell Biol.* **97:** 542.

———. 1989. The motor for poleward chromosome movement in anaphase is in or near the kinetochore. *J. Cell Biol.* **109:** 2245.

Oshimura, M. and J.C. Barrett. 1986. Chemical induced aneuploidy in mammalian cells: Mechanisms and biological significance in cancer. *Environ. Mutagen.* **8:** 129.

Oshimura, M., T.W. Hesterberg, and J.C. Barrett. 1986. An early, nonrandom karyotypic change in immortal Syrian hamster cell lines transformed by asbestos: Trisomy of chromosome 11. *Cancer Genet. Cytogenet.* **22:** 225.

Oshimura, M., T.W. Hesterberg, T. Tsutsui, and J.C. Barrett. 1984. Correlation of asbestos-induced cytogenetic effects with cell transformation of Syrian hamster embryo cells in culture. *Cancer Res.* **44:** 5017.

Palekar, L.D., J.F. Eyer, B.M. Most, and D.L. Coffin. 1987. Metaphase and anaphase analysis of V79 cells exposed to erionite, UICC chrysotile and UICC crocidolite. *Carcinogenesis* **8:** 553.

Pfarr, C.M., M. Cove, P.M. Grissom, T.S. Hays, M.E. Porter, and J.R. McIntosh. 1990. Cytoplasmic dynein is localized to kinetochores during mitosis. *Nature* **345:** 263.

Pluta, A.F., C.A. Cooke and W.C. Earnshaw. 1990. Structure of the human centromere at metaphase. *Trends Biochem. Sci.* **15:** 181.

Rappaport, R. 1986. Establishment of the mechanism of cytokinesis in animal cells. *Int. Rev. Cytol.* **101:** 245.

Rieder, C.L. 1982. The formation, structure and composition of the mammalian kinetochore and kinetochore fiber. *Int. Rev. Cytol.* **79:** 1.

———. 1990. Formation of the astral mitotic spindle: Ultrastructural basis for the centrosome-kinetochore interaction. *Electron Microsc. Rev.* **3:** 269.

Rieder, C.L. and S.P. Alexander. 1989. The attachment of chromosomes to the mitotic spindle and the production of aneuploidy in newt lung cells. In *Mechanisms of chromosome distribution and aneuploidy* (ed. M.A. Resnick and B.K. Vig), p. 185. A.R. Liss, New York.

———. 1990. Kinetochores are transported poleward along a single astral microtubule during chromosome attachment to the spindle in newt lung cells. *J. Cell Biol.* **110:** 81.

Rieder, C.L. and G.G. Borisy. 1982. The centrosome cycle in PtK2 cells: Asymmetric distribution and structural changes in the pericentriolar material. *Biol. Cell* **44:** 117.

Rieder, C.L. and R. Hard. 1990. Newt lung epithelial cells: Cultivation, use and advantages for biomedical research. *Int. Rev. Cytol.* **122:** 153.

Rieder, C.L., E.A. Davison, L.C.W. Jensen, L. Cassimeris, and E.D. Salmon. 1986. Oscillatory movements of monooriented chromosomes and their position relative to the spindle pole result from the ejection properties of the aster and half spindle. *J. Cell Biol.* **103:** 581.

Salmon, E.D. 1989a. Cytokinesis in animal cells. *Curr. Opin. Cell Biol.* **1:** 541.

———. 1989b. Microtubule dynamics and chromosome movement. In *Mitosis: Molecules and mechanisms* (ed. J. Hyams and B.R. Brinkley), p. 118. Academic Press, New York.

———. 1989c. Metaphase chromosome congression and anaphase poleward movement. In *Cell movement*, vol. 2. *Kinesin, dynein and microtubule dynamics* (ed. F.D. Warner and J.R. McIntosh), p.431. A.R. Liss, New York.

Sluder, G. 1979. Role of spindle microtubules in the control of cell cycle timing. *J. Cell Biol.* **80:** 674.

———. 1988. Control mechanisms of mitosis: The role of spindle microtubules in the timing of mitotic events. *Zool. Sci.* **5:** 653.

———. 1990a. Experimental analysis of centrosome reproduction in Echinoderm eggs. *Adv. Cell. Biol.* **3:** 221.

———. 1990b. Functional properties of kinetochores in animal cells. *Curr. Opin. Cell Biol.* **2:** 23.

Sluder, G. and D.A. Begg. 1983. Control mechanisms of the cell cycle: Role of the spatial arrangement of spindle components in the timing of mitotic events. *J. Cell Biol.* **97:** 877.

———. 1985. Experimental analysis of the reproduction of spindle poles. *J. Cell Sci.* **76:** 35.

Stanton, M.F., M. Layard, A. Tegeris, E. Miller, M. May, E. Morgan, and A. Smith. 1981. Relation of particle dimension to carcinogenicity in amphibole asbestos and other fibrous minerals. *J. Natl. Cancer Inst.* **67:** 965.

Steuer, E.R., L. Wordeman, T.A. Schroer, and M.P. Sheetz. 1990. Localization of cytoplasmic dynein to mitotic spindles and kinetochores. *Nature* **345:** 266.

Suzuki, Y. 1974. Interaction of asbestos with alveolar cells. *Environ. Health Perspect.* **9:** 241.

Suzuki, Y., J. Churg, and T. Ono. 1972. Phagocytic activity of the alveolar epithelial cells in pulmonary asbestosis. *Am. J. Pathol.* **69:** 373.

Sybenga, J. 1972. *General cytogenetics.* Elsevier, New York.

Topping, C.D. and P. Nettesheim. 1980. Two-stage carcinogenesis studies with asbestos in Fischer 344 rats. *J. Natl. Cancer Inst.* **65:** 627.

Vandre, D.D. and G.G. Borisy. 1989. The centrosome cycle in animal cells. In *Mitosis: Molecules and mechanisms* (ed. J. Hyams and B.R. Brinkley). p. 39. Academic Press, New York.

Wagner, J.C., G. Berry, J.W.S. Skidmore, and V. Timbrell. 1974. The effects of the inhalation of asbestos in rats. *Br. J. Cancer* **29:** 252.

Wang, N.S., M.C. Jaurand, L. Magne, L. Kheuang, M.C. Pinchon, and J. Bignon. 1987. The interactions between asbestos fibers and metaphase chromosomes of rat pleural mesothelial cells in culture. *Am. J. Pathol.* **126:** 343.

Weisburger, J.H. and G.M. Williams. 1981. Carcinogen testing: Current problems and new approaches. *Science* **214:** 401.

Wheatley, D.N. 1982. The centriole: A central enigma of cell biology. Elsevier, New York.

Zirkle, R.E. 1970a. Involvement of the prometaphase kinetochore in prevention of precocious anaphase. *J. Cell Biol.* **47:** 235a.

———. 1970b. UV-microbeam irradiation of newt-cell cytoplasm: Spindle destruction, false anaphase, and delay of true anaphase. *Radiation Res.* **41:** 516.

Role of Chromosomal Mutations in Asbestos-induced Cell Transformation

J.C. Barrett

Laboratory of Molecular Carcinogenesis, National Institute of Environmental Health Sciences, Research Triangle Park, North Carolina 27709

INTRODUCTION

Asbestos and other mineral dusts are carcinogenic to humans and animals (IARC 1977; National Research Council 1984), inducing predominantly two types of cancers: mesotheliomas and bronchogenic carcinomas. We have reviewed previously (Barrett et al. 1989) the evidence that asbestos is a complete carcinogen, an initiator, and a tumor promoter, indicating multiple mechanisms of action. Any single biological activity of asbestos fibers is therefore unlikely to be sufficient to explain the carcinogenic activity of this class of carcinogen. Unlike most other carcinogens, asbestos fibers are not directly electrophilic, do not form adducts with DNA, are inactive in the Ames *Salmonella* test, and fail to induce mutations at specific genetic loci in mammalian cells (Chamberlain and Tarmy 1977; Barrett 1987; Jaurand 1989). Some investigators have proposed therefore that asbestos is carcinogenic because of its tumor-promoting activity. This explanation, however, fails to explain fully the carcinogenic activity of mineral dusts (Barrett et al. 1989).

Although asbestos is not active as a gene mutagen in a variety of test systems, there is now clear evidence that it induces chromosomal mutations (aneuploidy and aberrations) in a wide variety of mammalian cells, including mesothelial cells (Lavappa et al. 1975; Sincock and Seabright 1975; Chamberlain and Tarmy 1977; Babu et al. 1980; Valerio et al. 1980; Oshimura et al. 1984; Lechner et al. 1985a,b; Jaurand et al. 1986; Barrett 1987; Jaurand 1989). It has also been shown that asbestos can induce transformation of cells in culture, including mesothelial cells and fibroblasts (Hesterberg and Barrett 1984; Hesterberg et al. 1986a; Lechner et al. 1985a; Patérour et al. 1985a,b). As will be discussed below, evidence exists with these model systems that the mechanism of asbestos-induced cell transformation involves a chromosomal mutation (Oshimura et al. 1984; Lechner et al. 1985a; Patérour et al. 1985a,b). In this paper, I focus on the mechanisms of mineral-fiber-induced cell transformation and chromosomal mutations and the significance of these effects to the carcinogenic mechanisms of these substances.

ASBESTOS-INDUCED CELL TRANSFORMATION

Although asbestos is inactive as a gene mutagen in mammalian cells (Jaurand 1989), it is able to induce heritable alterations in the growth properties of normal cells in culture. Lechner and co-workers (Lechner et al. 1985a,b) reported that asbestos alters the growth properties of human mesothelial cells and that this is associated with chromosomal changes in the treated cells. Jaurand and co-workers (Patérour et al. 1985a,b; Jaurand et al. 1986) have also shown that asbestos induces transformation and chromosomal changes in rat mesothelial cells in culture. Extensive studies from our laboratory have shown that asbestos and other mineral dusts induce neoplastic transformation of Syrian hamster embryo cells in culture. These investigations have provided possible insights into the mechanism of mineral dust carcinogenicity and the role of fiber dimensions on this process. These studies are discussed below in more detail.

The Syrian hamster embryo cell transformation assay has a number of advantages for studies of chemical carcinogenesis (Barrett et al. 1984, 1985). The cells in culture exhibit a low frequency of spontaneous transformation, but when treated with a wide variety of known carcinogens, the cells exhibit morphologic and growth alterations. These alterations (termed morphologic transformation) can be used as a quantitative assay for carcinogens. These alterations are induced by a wide variety of chemical carcinogens but not structurally related noncarcinogens. Of particular interest is the observation that this assay detects a number of known carcinogens that are frequently not detected in other short-term assays (e.g., asbestos, hormones, arsenic, benzene, and diethylhexylphtalate) (Barrett et al. 1985). Carcinogen-induced neoplastic transformation of these cells in culture is a multistep process, and this model can be used to study the intermediate steps in the carcinogenic process (Barrett and Ts'o 1978).

We observed that chrysotile and crocidolite asbestos induce a morphologic transformation of Syrian hamster embryo cells that is indistinguishable from cell transformation induced by other carcinogens, such as benzo(a)pyrene (Hesterberg and Barrett 1984). These investigations show that morphologically transformed cells progress and become tumorigenic after multiple passages, again similar to the findings with other carcinogens (Barrett and Ts'o 1978). The frequency of morphologically transformed cells increases linearly with increasing doses of asbestos (Fig. 1). Three other laboratories also have shown that asbestos fibers transform Syrian hamster embryo cells in culture (DiPaolo et al. 1983; Mikalsen et al. 1988; A. Tu, pers. comm.). Asbestos fibers can also transform BALB/c-3T3 cells in culture (Lu et al. 1988).

One of the more important (and intriguing) factors that influence mineral dust carcinogenicity is fiber dimension. Stanton et al. (1981) have shown in classical experiments that the mesothelioma-inducing activity of mineral dusts is related to fiber size, i.e., that thin fibers are more active than short, thick fibers. Similar to the induction of mesotheliomas in vivo, cell transformation in vitro by mineral fibers is dependent on fiber size (Hesterberg and Barrett 1984). Milling of chrysotile asbestos destroys its transforming activity, but this treatment reduces fiber diameter and fiber length. To study fiber length directly, the transformation by fiberglass was examined. Code 100 fiberglass (mean dia. = 0.1 μm) is more active than thicker code 110 fiberglass (mean dia. = 0.8 μm). Code 100 fiberglass (average length = 9.5 μm) is as equally potent as crocidolite asbestos of a similar length (Hesterberg and Barrett 1984). Milling of the code 100 fiberglass reduces the fiber length without affecting the fiber diameter. Reduction of fiber length to 2.2 μm reduces the transforming activity by 10- to 20-fold, and further reduction to <1 μm in length eliminates the transforming

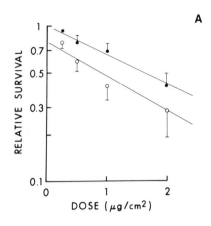

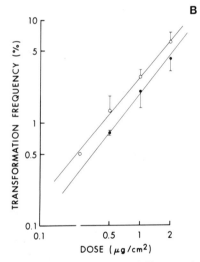

FIGURE 1 Effects of different doses of chrysotile (open circles) and crocidolite (closed circles) asbestos on the relative survival (A) and the morphologic transformation frequency of (B) Syrian hamster embryo cells in culture. Bars, S.E. (Reprinted, with permission, from Hesterberg and Barrett 1984.)

activity at the doses tested (Fig. 2). Thus, the fiber-length dependence of cell transformation parallels the results of mesothelioma induction in vivo.

The effects of other mineral dusts were also examined in

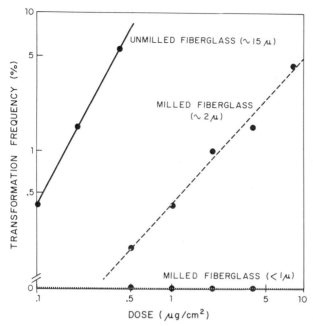

FIGURE 2 Effects of different doses of unmilled code 100 glass fibers (solid line) or milled code 100 (dashed line) on transformation frequency of Syrian hamster embryo cells in culture. (Reprinted, with permission, from Hesterberg and Barrett 1984.)

this transformation model. Min-U-Sil, a microcrystalline silica, is active but only at doses significantly greater than asbestos or fiberglass fibers. α-Quartz, another crystalline silica sample, is also active but only at higher doses. Interestingly, neither sample is very toxic, as measured by reduction in the colony-forming efficiencies of the treated cells.

To explore the mechanism of the asbestos-induced cell transformation, we examined the mutagenic effects of asbestos fibers in the same cell system (Oshimura et al. 1984). Consistent with other studies with mammalian cells, we found that asbestos fibers did not induce gene mutations in the cells under conditions that induce cell transformation. In contrast, asbestos fibers did induce chromosomal abnormalities in the treated cells, and the production of chromosomal mutations correlated with the transforming activity of the different fiber types. Chromosome mutations induced by the fiberglass are fiber-length dependent. The mineral fibers induce numerical chromosome changes; aneuploid cells both in the near-diploid range and in the tetraploid range are induced. Structural chromosome observations were also induced but only at low levels. The induction of aneuploidy appears to be the most significant chromosome change in the transformation process. This conclusion is based on the finding of a nonrandom chromosome change, an extra copy of chromosome 11, in the transformed cells (Oshimura et al. 1986). Trisomy 11 is the sole karyotypic change found in some of the asbestos-induced cell lines (Fig. 3).

We have proposed a mechanism for asbestos-induced aneuploidy, i.e., losses and gains of individual chromosomes (Hesterberg et al. 1986b). In collaboration with Dr. Arnold Brody,

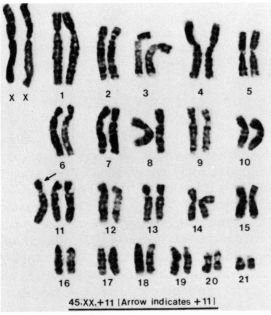

45,XX,+11 [Arrow indicates +11]

FIGURE 3 G-banded karyotype showing trisomy of chromosome 11 in the asbestos-induced Syrian hamster embryo 10W cell line. (Arrow) The extra chromosome. (Reprinted, with permission, from Oshimura and Barrett 1985.)

we showed that crocidolite asbestos fibers are taken up by the cells within 24 hours after treatment by phagocytosis (Hesterberg et al. 1986b); the intracellular fibers accumulate around the perinuclear region of the cells 24–48 hours after exposure (Fig. 4). When the cells undergo mitosis, the physical presence of the fibers results in interference with chromosome segregation.

Analysis of chrysotile-exposed cells in anaphase (Hesterberg and Barrett 1985) reveals a large increase in the number of cells with anaphase abnormalities including lagging chromosomes, bridges, and sticky chromosomes (Fig. 5). Asbestos fibers are observed in the mitotic cells and appear, in some cases, to interact directly with the chromosomes. Using ultrastructural analysis, Wang et al. (1987) have observed asbestos fibers apparently interacting with metaphase chromosomes after treatment of rat mesothelial cells in culture. From these studies, we propose that the physical interaction of the asbestos fibers with the chromosomes or structural proteins of the spindle apparatus causes missegregation of chromosomes during mitosis, resulting in aneuploidy. These findings provide a mechanism, at the chromosomal level, by which asbestos and other mineral fibers might induce cell transformation and cancer. Malignant human and rat mesotheliomas are highly aneuploid (Gibas et al. 1986; Stenman et al. 1986). It is possible that asbestos exposure leads to the generation of these aneuploid cells in vivo as well as in vitro.

Nonfibrous particles, such as silica, are also phagocytized by the cells and accumulate on the perinuclear region (Hesterberg et al. 1986a). The presence of these particles at mitosis also results in aneuploidy induction but at higher doses than required for fibrous minerals. The cells can accumulate large numbers of silica particles without cytotoxicity, transformation, or aneuploidy induction.

Two factors appear to contribute to the fiber-size dependence of asbestos-induced cell transformation and chromosome damage. Hesterberg et al. (1986b) quantitated the number of intracellular fibers in Syrian hamster embryo cells exposed to long and short fiberglass. The phagocytosis and intracellular distribution of glass fibers of differing lengths were examined at various times after treatment. The average length

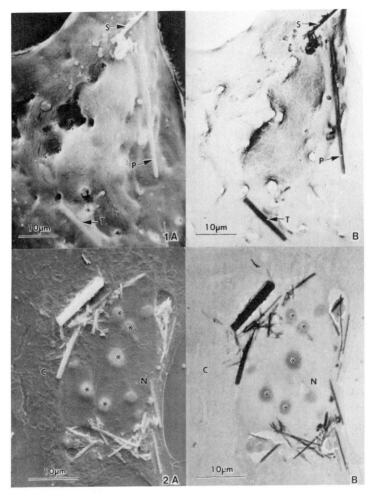

FIGURE 4 Scanning electron micrographs (*1A, 2A*) and the corresponding backscatter electron images (*1B, 2B*), showing the perinuclear accumulation of crocidolite asbestos fibers by a Syrian hamster embryo cell 24 hr after treatment with 1 μg/cm². Nuclear region (*N*) is demarcated by prominent nucleoli (asterisks). (C) Cytoplasm. Magnification, 1525x. (Reprinted, with permission, from Hesterberg et al. 1986b.)

of the fibers that are phagocytized is greater than the average length of the fibers exposed to the cells. This indicates that cells phagocytize longer fibers more effectively than shorter

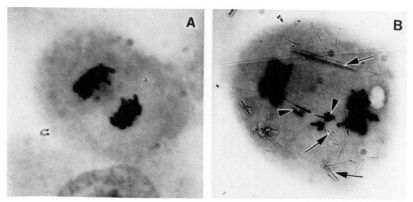

FIGURE 5 Normal (A) and an abnormal (B) anaphase from crocidolite-asbestos-treated Syrian hamster embryo cells. Note the asbestos fibers (arrows), some of which appear to be associated with displaced chromosomes (arrowheads) in the abnormal anaphase. (Reprinted, with permission, from Hesterberg and Barrett 1985.)

fibers. In our experiment that was designed to compare the uptake of fibers of different lengths, glass-fiber length was decreased from approximately 15 µm to approximately 2 µm by milling with a mortar and pestle, and cells were treated with an equal dose (1 µg/cm^2) of milled or unmilled fibers. Since fiber length was reduced sevenfold in the milled sample, the cells were exposed to sevenfold more fibers with the milled sample. However, cells exposed to the milled fiberglass had a similar number of fibers per cell as those exposed to unmilled fibers. This again indicates that the shorter fibers are less readily phagocytized. Thus, fiber length affects intracellular fiber accumulation. Fiber length, however, did not appear to affect the migration of intracellular fibers to the perinuclear region of the cytoplasm. Even though cells treated with milled glass fibers contained a similar number of fibers as those treated with unmilled glass fibers, the resulting cytotoxicity, transformation frequency, and frequency of micronuclei were greatly reduced in the cultures treated with milled glass fibers. Thus, fiber length appears to affect the phagocytosis of fibers, as well as the ability of intracellular fibers to induce cytogenetic damage and the resultant transformation.

ROLE OF FIBER-INDUCED CHROMOSOMAL CHANGES IN ASBESTOS-RELATED CANCERS

One approach to elucidating the mechanisms of asbestos car-cinogenicity is to define the critical molecular alterations in asbestos-induced cancers. Since mesotheliomas are induced predominately as the consequence of asbestos exposure, these are ideal cancers for this analysis. Karyotypic analyses of hu-man mesotheliomas (for review, see Barrett et al. 1991) reveal multiple chromosome changes. Chromosomes 1, 2, 3, 6, 11, 17, and 22 are most frequently involved in either numerical or structural rearrangements. Nonrandom deletions of multiple chromosomal regions are observed.

Asbestos and other mineral fibers induce multiple types of cancers and are likely to act by multiple mechanisms. Al-though asbestos fibers do not induce gene mutations, they are effective inducers of chromosome alterations. There is increas-ing evidence for the involvement of two classes of genes in car-cinogenesis, oncogenes and tumor suppressor genes. Onco-genes are the activated forms of a family of normal cellular genes, proto-oncogenes. These genes when activated by a vari-ety of mutational events, including point mutation, chromo-some translocation, and gene amplification, result in a posi-tive, proliferative signal for the cells. In contrast, tumor sup-pressor genes negatively regulate tumor cell growth and are frequently inactivated or lost in tumors. These genes are in-activated by chromosome loss, chromosome deletion, recombi-nation, and point mutations (Barrett and Wiseman 1987). Be-cause asbestos fibers fail to induce point mutations, they would not be expected to activate proto-oncogenes or to inacti-vate tumor suppressor genes by this mechanism. Asbestos-induced chromosome breaks may result in activation of proto-oncogenes. More likely, asbestos-induced chromosome loss or deletion could result in inactivation of tumor suppressor genes.

The identification in human mesothelioma of activated transforming genes (Barrett et al. 1989) and the loss of specific chromosomal regions (Barrett et al. 1991) are indicative that proto-oncogenes and tumor suppressor genes are altered in these cancers. It will be important in the future to understand the role of asbestos fibers in these alterations. A further understanding of the mechanism of action of asbestos should focus on addressing whether these genes are mutated directly or indirectly by fibers.

REFERENCES

Babu, K.A., B.C. Lakkad, S.K. Nigam, D.K. Bhatt, A.B. Karnik, K.N. Thakore, S.K. Kashyap, and S.K. Chatterjee. 1980. In vitro cytological and cytogenetic effects of an Indian variety of chrysotile asbestos. *Environ. Res.* **21:** 416.

Barrett, J.C., ed. 1987. Relationship between mutagenesis and carcinogenesis. In *Mechanisms of environmental carcinogenesis: Role of genetic and epigenetic changes,* vol. 1, p. 129. CRC Press, Boca Raton, Florida.

Barrett, J.C. and P.O.P. Ts'o. 1978. Evidence for the progressive nature of neoplastic transformation in vitro. *Proc. Natl. Acad. Sci.* **75:** 3761.

Barrett, J.C. and R.W. Wiseman. 1987. Cellular and molecular mechanisms of multistep carcinogenesis: Relevance of carcinogen risk assessment. *Environ. Health Perspect.* **76:** 65.

Barrett, J.C., T.W. Hesterberg, and D.G. Thomassen. 1984. Use of cell transformation systems for carcinogenicity testing and mechanistic studies of carcinogenesis. *Pharmacol. Rev.* **36:** 53S.

Barrett, J.C., P.W. Lamb, and R.W. Wiseman. 1989. Multiple mechanisms for the carcinogenic effects of asbestos and other mineral fibers. *Environ. Health Perspect.* **81:** 81.

Barrett, J.C., C. Walker, and J. Everitt. 1991. Possible cellular and molecular mechanisms for asbestos carcinogenicity. *Am. J. Ind. Med.* (in press).

Barrett, J.C., T.W. Hesterberg, M. Oshimura, and T. Tsutsui. 1985. Role of chemically induced mutagenic events in neoplastic transformation of Syrian hamster embryo cells. *Carcinog. Compr. Surv.* **9:** 123.

Chamberlain, M. and E.M. Tarmy. 1977. Asbestos and glass fibers in bacterial mutation tests. *Mutat. Res.* **43:** 159.

DiPaolo, J.A., A.J. DeMarinis, and J. Doniger. 1983. Asbestos and benzo(a)pyrene synergism in the transformation of Syrian hamster embryo cells. *Pharmacology* **27:** 65.

Gibas, Z., F.P. Li, K.H. Antman, S. Bernai, R. Stahel, and A.A. Sandberg. 1986. Chromosome changes in malignant mesothelioma. *Cancer Genet. Cytogenet.* **20:** 191.

Hesterberg, T.W. and J.C. Barrett. 1984. Dependence of asbestos- and mineral dust-induced transformation of mammalian cells in culture on fiber dimension. *Cancer Res.* **44:** 2170.

————. 1985. Induction by asbestos fibers of anaphase abnormalities: Mechanism for aneuploidy induction and possibly carcinogenesis. *Carcinogenesis* **6:** 473.

Hesterberg, T.W., A.R. Brody, M. Oshimura, and J.C. Barrett. 1986a. Asbestos and silica induce morphological transformation of mammalian cells in culture: A possible mechanism. In *Silica, silicosis, and cancer* (ed. D.F. Goldsmith et al.), p. 177. Praeger Press, New York.

Hesterberg, T.W., C.J. Butterick, M. Oshimura, A.R. Brody, and J.C. Barrett. 1986b. Role of phagocytosis in Syrian hamster cell transformation and cytogenetic effects induced by asbestos and short and long glass fibers. *Cancer Res.* **46:** 5795.

IARC. 1977. Asbestos. *IARC Monogr. Eval. Carcinog. Risk Chem. Hum.* **14.**

Jaurand, M.C. 1989. A particulate state carcinogenesis: Recent data on the mechanisms of action of fibers. *IARC Publ.* **90:** 54.

Jaurand, M.C., L. Kheuang, L. Magne, and J. Bignon. 1986. Chromosomal changes induced by chrysotile fibers or benzo-3,4-pyrene in rat pleural mesothelial cells. *Mutat. Res.* **169:** 141.

Lavappa, K.S., M.M. Fu, and S.S. Epstein. 1975. Cytogenetic studies on chrysotile asbestos. *Environ. Res.* **10:** 165.

Lechner, J.F., T. Tokiwa, H. Yeager, Jr., and C.C. Harris. 1985a. Associated chromosomal changes in human mesothelial cells. *NATO ASI Ser. G Ecol. Sci.* **3:** 197.

Lechner, J.F., T. Tokiwa, M. LaVeck, W.F. Benedict, S. Banks-Schlegel, H. Yeager, Jr., A. Banerjee, and C.C. Harris. 1985b. Asbestos-associated chromosomal changes in human mesothelial cells. *Proc. Natl. Acad. Sci.* **82:** 3884.

Lu, Y.-P., C. Lasne, R. Lowy, and I. Chouroulinkov. 1988. Use of the orthogonal design method to study the synergistic effects of asbestos fibers and 12-*O*-tetradecanoylphorbol-13-acetate (TPA) in the BALB/3T3 cell transformation system. *Mutagenesis* **3:** 355.

Mikalsen, S.O., E. Rivedal, and T. Sanner. 1988. Morphological transformation of Syrian hamster embryo cells induced by mineral fibres and the alleged enhancement of benzo(a)pyrene. *Carcinogenesis* **9:** 891.

National Research Council. 1984. *Asbestiform fibers: Nonoccupational health risks.* National Academy Press, Washington, D.C.

Oshimura, M. and J.C. Barrett. 1985. Double nondisjunction during karyotypic progression of chemically induced Syrian hamster cell lines. *Cancer Genet. Cytogenet.* **18:** 131.

Oshimura, M., T.W. Hesterberg, and J.C. Barrett. 1986. An early, nonrandom karyotypic change in immortal Syrian hamster cell lines transformed by asbestos: Trisomy of chromosome 11. *Cancer Genet. Cytogenet.* **22:** 225.

Oshimura, M., T.W. Hesterberg, T. Tsutsui, and J.C. Barrett. 1984. Correlation of asbestos-induced cytogenetic effects with cell transformation of Syrian hamster embryo cells in culture. *Cancer Res.* **44:** 5017.

Patérour, M.J., J. Bignon, and M.C. Jaurand. 1985a. *In vitro* transformation of rat pleural mesothelial cells by chrysotile and/or benzo(a) pyrene. *Carcinogenesis* **6:** 523.

Patérour, M.J., A. Renier, J. Bignon, and M.C. Jaurand. 1985b. Induction of transformation in cultured rat pleural mesothelial cells by chrysotile fibers. *NATO ASI. Ser. Ser. G Ecol. Sci.* **3:** 203.

Sincock, A.M. and M. Seabright. 1975. Induction of chromosome changes in Chinese hamster cells by exposure to asbestos fibers. *Nature* **257:** 56.

Stanton, M.F., M. Layard, A. Tegeris, E. Miller, M. May, E. Morgan, and A. Smith. 1981. Relation of particle dimension to carcinogenicity in amphibole asbestoses and other fibrous minerals. *J. Natl. Cancer Inst.* **67:** 965.

Stenman, C., K. Olofsson, T. Mansson, B. Hagmar, and J. Mark. 1986. Chromosomes and chromosomal evolution in human mesotheliomas as reflected in sequential analyses of two cases. *Hereditas* **105:** 233.

Valerio, F., M. DeFerran, L. Ottaggio, E. Repetto, and L. Santi. 1980. Cytogenetic effects of Rhodesian chrysotile on human lymphocytes *in vitro. IARC Sci. Publ.* **1:** 485.

Wang, N.S., M.C. Jaurand, L. Magne, L. Kheuang, M.C. Pinchon, and J. Bignon. 1987. The interactions between asbestos fibers and metaphase chromosomes of rat pleural mesothelial cells in culture. *Am. J. Pathol.* **126:** 343.

Cytogenetics of Human Mesothelioma

M. Tiainen,[1] L. Tammilehto,[2] J. Rautonen,[3] K. Mattson,[2] and S. Knuutila[1]

[1]Department of Medical Genetics, University of Helsinki, Haartmaninkatu 3
00290 Helsinki, Finland
[2]Department of Pulmonary Medicine, University of Helsinki
Haartmaninkatu 4, 00290 Helsinki, Finland
[3]Department of Pediatrics, University of Helsinki, Stenbäckinatu 11, 00290
Helsinki, Finland

INTRODUCTION

The incidence of malignant mesothelioma, a mesodermally derived tumor, has increased with the growing use of asbestos in industry (Antman 1980; Browne 1986). The histological and cytological distinction between mesothelioma and adenocarcinoma metastatic to the pleura is not always clear (Battifora and Kopinski 1985; Burns et al. 1985). During the past few years, it has been widely accepted that chromosome study is an important tool with both clinical and biological significance in human neoplasms (Heim and Mitelman 1987). Since the existing information about chromosomal abnormalities in mesothelioma appeared very scanty (Heim and Mitelman 1987; Mitelman 1988), we undertook to analyze the chromosomes of fresh tumor cells from patients with malignant pleural mesothelioma. This summary of our studies (Tiainen et al. 1988, 1989) shows chromosomal abnormalities in malignant mesothelioma to be nonrandom and of prognostic importance. Some of the recurrent abnormalities appear to correlate with high asbestos exposure.

PATIENTS AND METHODS

The diagnosis and histological subtyping of the mesotheliomas were confirmed by two independent pathology panels: the Finnish National Mesothelioma Pathology Panel and the Mesothe-

Cellular and Molecular Aspects of Fiber Carcinogenesis
Copyright 1991 Cold Spring Harbor Laboratory Press 0-87969-361-4/91 $1.00 + 00

lioma Pathology Panel of the Lung Cancer Cooperative Group of the European Organization for Research and Treatment of Cancer. A total of 38 patients were studied. Of these, 30 were men and 8 were women. The mean age at diagnosis was 59 years (range, 39–83 years). The histological subtype was epithelial in 19 patients, mixed in 16, and fibromatous in 2. In one patient, the specimen available allowed cytological diagnosis but no histological subtyping. Chromosome-G-banding analysis of metaphase chromosomes, according to the methods of Tiainen et al. (1988), was performed on cells of fresh tumor specimens from 32 patients (37 specimens) and/or on cells isolated from the pleural fluid of 27 patients (38 specimens). Both specimens were available from 21 patients. Specimens were obtained before treatment from 32 patients.

Asbestos exposure was evaluated in 16 patients by determining the content of asbestos fibers in samples of dried lung tissue (Tuomi et al. 1989). Of these patients, 11 had >5 million asbestos fibers per gram in their lung tissue (range, 5.5–370 million fibers/g). They had been exposed to asbestos while employed in shipbuilding, building construction, and maintenance. Five patients had <5 million fibers per gram of lung tissue (range, 0.1–3.1 million fibers/g). They had been exposed to asbestos while employed in the construction industry, electrical installation work, powerplants, and transportation. The main asbestos fiber types found in both groups were crocidolite, amosite, and anthophyllite. The latency period between the exposure and diagnosis of mesothelioma was very long in the majority of the patients, and the work during which the exposure was considered to have taken place had in most cases continued for several years (Tuomi et al. 1989).

The patients' treatment consisted of multimodality therapy encompassing debulking surgery, chemotherapy, and hemithorax irradiation. The chemotherapy was either single-agent therapy with mitoxantrone or epirubicin or combination therapy with cyclophosphamide, vincristin, doxorubicin, and dakarbazin (CYVADIC). Three different time-dose-fractionation programs of hemithorax irradiation were applied (Holsti and Mattson 1988). More detailed patient characteristics, individual therapies, and survival data were presented previously by Tiainen et al. (1988, 1989).

RESULTS

Success Rate: Metaphases for Banding Analysis

Mitotic cells for chromosome-banding analysis were obtained from 34 of 38 patients and from 56 of 75 specimens (24 of 37 tumors and 32 out of 38 effusion fluids).

Chromosomal Aneuploidy

Clonal chromosomal aneuploidy was observed in 25 of 34 patients: 21 patients had a pseudodiploid or near-diploid chromosome number (13 patients also had polyploid variants of the near-diploid clone), and 4 patients had a triploid-tetraploid clone. Most of the patients also had cells with normal karyotype and cells with nonclonal abnormalities. A chromosomal abnormality was classified as clonal if it appeared in at least two cells, except in the case of chromosomal loss where the chromosomal abnormality's presence was required in at least three cells. A detailed description of the abnormalities was presented previously (Tiainen et al. 1988, 1989).

With the exception of three specimens, all 25 patients exhibited very complex karyotype abnormalities (Fig. 1). The karyotypes of the exceptional specimens were 48,XX,+5,+7 (patient no. 16), 46,XY,t(9;11)/+21,t(14q;17q)/t(5;13) (three different clones, patient no. 31), and 50,XY,+X,+Y,+i(5p),+i(5p) (patient no. 36). In addition, patients 6 and 8 had simple clones (45,XY,–Y and 47,XY,+Y, respectively) in some specimens but quite different clones involving complex chromosomal abnormalities in other specimens that were obtained from the same tumors before treatment. It is possible that in patients 16, 31, and 36, as well as in the 9 patients with normal karyotypes and/or nonclonal abnormalities, complex clones were also present, although they were undetected in the cytogenetic analysis. In addition to the extreme complexity of the abnormalities, several sublines were observed, indicating clonal evolution.

Structural Chromosome Abnormalities

A wide range of structural aberrations, such as deletions, isochromosomes, and unbalanced translocations, were seen.

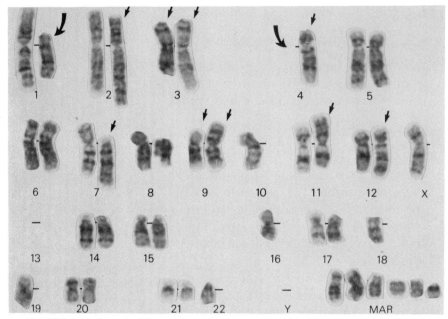

FIGURE 1 G-banded karyotype from patient 13 (Tiainen et al. 1988) involving several structural chromosomal aberrations (small arrows). Breakpoint at 1p11, partial monosomy 1, and monosomy 4 (large arrows) were associated with a high concentration of asbestos fibers in lung tissue, which in this patient was 370 million fibers per gram of dried tissue.

In addition, double-minute chromosomes, homogeneously staining regions, and endoreduplication phenomena were observed. In general, breakpoints were encountered in all chromosomes except 18 and Y (Fig. 2). Most breakpoints occurred in chromosomes 1, 3, 2, 9, 11, and 7, in decreasing order of frequency. It is worth noting that a distinct hot spot seemed to be located in the p-arm of chromosome 1 (Fig. 2).

Numerical Chromosome Abnormalities

The most frequent numerical abnormalities were partial or total monosomy 22 (14 patients), monosomy 1 (12 patients), monosomy 3 (12 patients), monosomy 9 (11 patients), partial or total polysomy 7 (13 patients), and polysomy 11 (11 patients). In addition, monosomy of chromosomes 4, 14, and

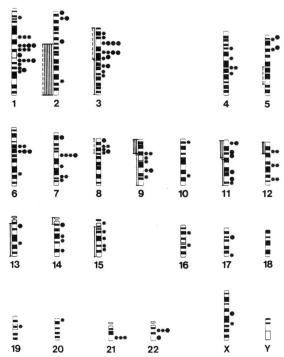

FIGURE 2 Distribution of chromosomal breakpoints in cases with clonal abnormalities. Each asterisk and each line (patients nos. 1, 3, 5, 6, 8, 9, 10, 12, 13, 14, 16, 17, 18, 21, 23, 25, 26, 27, and 29 [Tiainen et al. 1988]) and each dot and each dotted line (patients nos. 20, 31, 32, 33, 35, and 36 [Tiainen et al. 1989]) represent one breakpoint (lines indicate breakpoints that could not be determined exactly). Reprinted, with permission, from Tiainen et al. (1989).

15 and polysomy of chromosomes 5 and 12 were frequently observed.

Chromosome Abnormalities Reported in the Literature

To our knowledge, only a few cytogenetic reports concerning about 80 patients with malignant mesothelioma can be found in the literature (Mark 1978; Gibas et al. 1986; Stenman et al. 1986; Bello et al. 1987; Popescu et al. 1988; Flejter et al. 1989; Hagemeijer et al. 1990; Pelin-Enlund et al. 1990). Most of these studies have included pleural effusions or cell lines instead of primary tumor specimens. The results appear mainly to coincide with our results of primary tumors and pleural effusions from 38 patients. Hagemeijer et al. (1990) have also found chromosomes 1, 3, 4, 5, 6, 9, 10, 20, and 22 to be recurrently affected. These investigators observed gains of chromosomes 7 and 11 less frequently than we did. Flejter et al. (1989) compiled data on 25 patients from the literature, including some of our patients and 5 patients of their own. Their compiled series confirmed a recurrent breakpoint in chromosome 1p and aneuploidy in chromosomes 3, 4, 7, 14, and 22.

Coexistence of Different Chromosomal Abnormalities

When our data were tested for coexistence of different chromosomal abnormalities (Tiainen et a. 1989), two groups could be discerned: a group of chromosome gains, including polysomy 7, and a group of chromosomal losses, including loss of chromosome 3 and/or breakpoint 1p11–p22 (Fig. 3). Such correlations might indicate cooperation of different oncogenes or growth factor genes and loss of tumor suppressor genes. It is interesting that N-*ras* or two N-*ras*-like oncogenes, as well as epidermal growth factor receptor gene (*erbB* oncogene homolog), methionine (*met*) oncogene, platelet-derived growth factor genes (PDGFA and PDGFB), and P-glycoprotein genes 1 and 3 (*mdr1* and *mdr3* [multidrug resistance]), have all been localized to chromosomes 1, 7, 9, and 22 (McAlpine et al. 1989).

Polysomy 7 and Survival

Apart from polysomy 7, other abnormalities did not show any correlation with survival. There was a statistically significant correlation ($p = 0.02$) between prognosis and the number of copies of the p-arm of chromosome 7. The more there were copies of 7p present, the shorter was the survival (Fig. 4).

Correlation of Chromosome Abnormalities with Asbestos Fiber Burden

For the study of a correlation between chromosome abnormalities and the content of asbestos fibers in lung tissue (Tuomi et

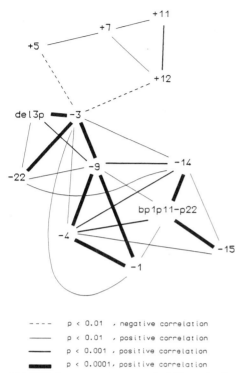

- - - -	p < 0.01 , negative correlation
———	p < 0.01 , positive correlation
———	p < 0.001 , positive correlation
▬▬▬	p < 0.0001, positive correlation

FIGURE 3 Coexistence of different chromosome abnormalities. (–/+) Partial or total chromosome loss or gain; (del3p) deletion of the p-arm of chromosome 3; (bp1p11–p22) breakpoint at 1p11–p22. Reprinted, with permission, from Tiainen et al. (1989).

al. 1989), specimens from 16 patients were divided into two groups: a low-asbestos-content group and a high-asbestos-content group, with 5 million fibers per gram as the dividing point.

Out of the 16 patients, 11 who were studied belonged to the high-asbestos-content group with concentrations between 5.5 million and 370 million fibers per gram of dried lung tissue. Partial or total loss of chromosomes 1 and 4 or breakpoint 1p11–p22 correlated significantly with high asbestos content in lung tissue (Fig. 1, $p = 0.0001$, $p = 0.003$, $p = 0.009$, respectively).

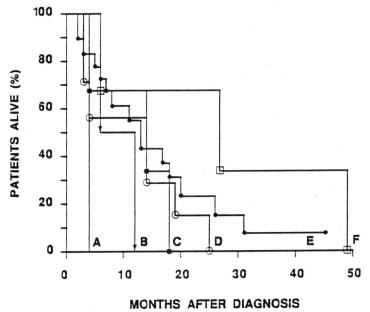

MONTHS AFTER DIAGNOSIS

FIGURE 4 Correlation between survival and the number of copies of the p-arm of chromosome 7 (p = 0.02). (*A*) Four extra p-arms (patient no. 29); (*B*) three extra p-arms (patients nos. 8 and 10); (*C*) two extra p-arms (patients nos. 17, 21, and 23); (*D*) one extra 7p (patients nos. 6, 9, 14, 16, 18, 26, and 33); (*E*) normal number of p-arms (patients nos. 1, 2, 4, 5, 11, 12, 15, 19, 20, 22, 24, 25, 27, 31, 34, 35, 36, and 38); (*F*) loss of one p-arm (patients nos. 3, 13, and 32). Reprinted, with permission, from Tiainen et al. (1989).

COMMENTS

The results presented here demonstrate that most cases of malignant pleural mesothelioma are associated with clonal chromosome abnormalities. The abnormalities are generally very complex, exhibiting several subclones with both structural and numerical abnormalities. This indicates an advanced stage of the malignant process, which is in agreement with the poor prognosis seen in our patients and in those of other investigators (Antman 1980). None of the abnormalities reported here are specific for malignant mesothelioma and thus have no diagnostic value. Abnormalities in chromosomes 1, 3, 7, and 22 have been described in a wide range of solid tumors, including adenocarcinoma of the lung (Brito-Babapulle and Atkin 1981; Whang-Peng et al. 1982; Zang 1982; Balaban et al. 1986; Sandberg 1986; Fan and Li 1987; Kovacs et al. 1987; Rey et al. 1987; Bigner et al. 1988).

The complexity of the karyotypes makes it difficult to deduce primary chromosome changes. Structural aberrations involving a breakpoint at 1p11–p22 and partial or total monosomy of chromosomes 1 and 4 that were associated with asbestos exposure could be some of the primary abnormalities. On the other hand, there were three patients with a single or only a few abnormalities (e.g., gain of chromosome 5 and/or chromosome 7 material in two of them), which might be significant.

In addition to monosomy 22, loss of material from other chromosomes, especially chromosomes 1, 3, 4, and 9, was frequent in our cases and in those reported by other investigators (Flejter et al. 1989; Hagemeijer et al. 1990). This finding suggests that recessive cancer genes might be operative in the malignant transformation of mesothelial cells.

The correlations of polysomy 7 with poor prognosis and of breakpoint 1p11–p22 and partial or total loss of chromosomes 1 or 4 with asbestos fiber burden have not been studied so far by other investigators. The question of whether asbestos induces specific aberrations in chromosomes 1 and 4 warrants further study. There are, however, reports on rat mesotheliomas (Libbus and Graighead 1988), on Syrian hamster cell lines transformed by asbestos (Oshimura et al. 1986), and on human mesothelial cells exposed to asbestos (Lechner et al. 1985; Olofsson and Mark 1989) that suggest that asbestos may cause nonrandom karyotype changes.

In conclusion, it is obvious that cytogenetic study has clinical and biological significance in malignant mesothelioma. Karyotype analysis of metaphase chromosomes is, however, time consuming, and sometimes a successful analysis cannot be performed at all. Interphase cytogenetic analysis by means of in situ hybridization with chromosome-specific probes is a recent method that allows the study of chromosome aneuploidy in nondividing cells also (Rappold et al. 1984; Cremer et al. 1986; Hopman et al. 1988). Compared to karyotype analysis, interphase cytogenetics is relatively fast and easy to perform. It is also important that the study can be performed on

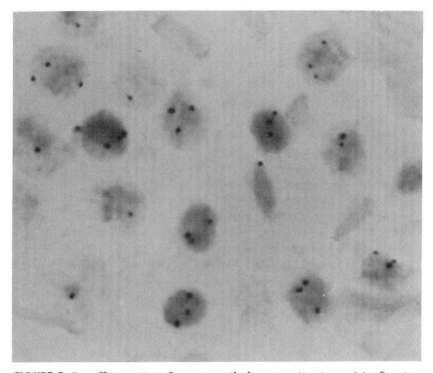

FIGURE 5 Paraffin section from mesothelioma patient no. 14 after in situ hybridization with chromosome-7-specific α-satellite DNA probe D7Z2 (p21-4, kindly provided by Dr. H.F. Willard). Numerous interphase nuclei with three hybridization signals were seen, coinciding with the result of the karyotype analysis with three copies of chromosome 7 (M. Tiainen et al., in prep.).

histologically, morphologically, and immunologically characterized cells (Wessman and Knuutila 1988; Emmerich et al. 1989). Thus, it is possible to study chromosome aberrations, for example, on large series of tumor samples even in pathological laboratories. More extensive series are needed before one can reliably assess the prognostic and biological importance of polysomy 7 and other frequent chromosomal abnormalities seen in malignant mesothelioma. We have used in situ hybridization techniques with chromosome-1- and chromosome-7-specific centrometric α-satellite DNA probes on paraffin-embedded sections of mesothelioma. Our preliminary results show that interphase cytogenetic analysis is suitable for studying numerical chromosome abnormalities in tumor specimens of malignant mesothelioma (Fig. 5), and more information is obtained compared with that derived from karyotype analysis (M. Tiainen et al., in prep.).

ACKNOWLEDGMENTS

This work was partly supported by grants from the Finnish Cancer Society and the Sigrid Juselius Foundation.

REFERENCES

Antman, K.H. 1980. Current concepts. Malignant mesothelioma. *N. Engl. J. Med.* **303**: 200.

Balaban, G.B., M. Herlyn, W.H. Clark, Jr., and P.C. Nowell. 1986. Karyotypic evolution in human malignant melanoma. *Cancer Genet. Cytogenet.* **19**: 113.

Battifora, H. and M.I. Kopinski. 1985. Distinction of mesothelioma from adenocarcinoma, an immunohistochemical approach. *Cancer* **55**: 1679.

Bello, M.J., J.A. Rey, M.J. Aviles, M. Arevalo, and J. Benitez. 1987. Cytogenetic findings in an effusion secondary from pleural mesothelioma. *Cancer Genet. Cytogenet.* **29**: 75.

Bigner, S.H., J. Mark, P.C. Burger, M.S. Mahaley, Jr., D.E. Bullard, L.H. Muhlbaier, and D.D. Bigner. 1988. Specific chromosomal abnormalities in malignant human gliomas. *Cancer Res.* **88**: 405.

Brito-Babapulle, V. and N.B. Atkin. 1981. Break points in chromosome 1 abnormalities of 218 human neoplasms. *Cancer Genet. Cytogenet.* **4**: 215.

Browne, K. 1986. Mesothelioma registry data. *Lancet* **I**: 167.

Burns, T.R., S.D. Greenberg, M.L. Mace, and E.H. Johnson. 1985. Ultrastructural diagnosis of epithelial malignant mesothelioma. *Cancer* **56**: 2036.

Cremer, T., J. Landegent, A. Brueckner, H.P. Scholl, M. Schardin, H.D. Hager, P. Devilee, P. Pearson, and M. van der Ploeg. 1986. Detection of chromosome aberrations in the human interphase nucleus by visualization of specific target DNAs with radioactive and non-radioactive in situ hybridization techniques: Diagnosis of trisomy 18 with probe L1.84. *Hum. Genet.* **74**: 346.

Emmerich, P., A. Jauch, M.C. Hofmann, T. Cremer, and H. Walt. 1989. Methods in laboratory investigation. Interphase cytogenetics in paraffin embedded sections from human testicular germ cell tumor xenografts and in corresponding cultured cells. *Lab. Invest.* **61:** 235.

Fan, Y.S. and P. Li. 1987. Cytogenetic studies of four human lung adenocarcinoma cell lines. *Cancer Genet. Cytogenet.* **26:** 317.

Flejter, W.L., F.P. Li, K.H. Antman, and J.R. Testa. 1989. Recurring loss involving chromosomes 1, 3, and 22 in malignant mesothelioma: Possible sites of tumor suppressor genes. *Genes Chrom. Cancer* **1:** 148.

Gibas, Z., F.P. Li, K.H. Antman, S. Bernal, R. Stahel, and A.A. Sandberg. 1986. Chromosome changes in malignant mesothelioma. *Cancer Genet. Cytogenet.* **20:** 191.

Hagemeijer, A., M.A. Versnel, E. Van Drunen, M. Moret, M.J. Bouts, T.H. van der Kwast, and H.C. Hoogsteden. 1990. Cytogenetic analysis of malignant mesothelioma. *Cancer Genet. Cytogenet.* **47:** 1.

Heim, S. and F. Mitelman. 1987. *Cancer cytogenetics.* A.R. Liss, New York.

Holsti, L.R. and K. Mattson. 1988. Hemithorax irradiation in the treatment of pleural mesothelioma. In *Proceedings of the 5th Varian European Clinac Users Meeting,* February 1987 (ed. A.B.M.F. Karin et al.), p. 166. Flims, Switzerland.

Hopman A.H.N., F.C.S. Ramaekers, A.K. Raap, J.L.M. Beck, P. Devilee, M. van der Ploeg, and G.P. Voojis. 1988. In situ hybridization as a tool to study numerical chromosome aberrations in solid bladder tumors. *Histochemistry* **89:** 307.

Kovacs, G., S. Szucs, W. De Riese, and H. Baumgärtel. 1987. Specific chromosome aberration in human renal cell carcinoma. *Int. J. Cancer* **40:** 171.

Lechner, J.F., T. Tokiwa, M. La Veck, W.F. Benedict, S. Banks-Schlegel, H. Yeager, A. Danerjee, and C.C. Harris. 1985. Asbestos-associated chromosomal changes in human mesothelial cells. *Proc. Natl. Acad. Sci.* **82:** 3884.

Libbus, B.L. and J.E. Graighead. 1988. Chromosomal translocations with specific breakpoints in asbestos-induced rat mesotheliomas. *Cancer Res.* **48:** 6348.

Mark, J. 1978. Monosomy 14, monosomy 22 and 13q-. Three chromosomal abnormalities observed in cells of two malignant mesotheliomas studied by banding techniques. *Acta Cytol.* **22:** 398.

McAlpine, P.J., T.B. Shows, C. Boucheix, L.C. Stranc, T.G. Berent, A.J. Pakstis, and R.C. Doute. 1989. Report of the nomenclature committee and the 1989 catalog of mapped genes. *Cytogenet. Cell Genet.* **51:** 13.

Mitelman, F. 1988. *Catalog of chromosome aberrations in cancer,* third edition. A.R. Liss, New York.

Olofsson, K. and J. Mark. 1989. Specificity of asbestos-induced chromosomal aberrations in short-term cultured human mesothelial cells. *Cancer Genet. Cytogenet.* **41:** 33.

Oshimura, M., T.W. Hesterberg, and J.C. Barret. 1986. An early nonrandom karyotypic change in immortal Syrian hamster cell lines transformed by asbestos: Trisomy of chromosome 11. *Cancer Genet. Cytogenet.* **22:** 225.

Pelin-Enlund, K., K. Husgavel-Pursiainen, L. Tammilehto, M. Klockars, K. Jantunen, B.I. Gerwin, C.C. Harris, T. Tuomi, E. Vanhala, K. Mattson, and K. Linnainmaa. 1990. Asbestos-related malignant mesothelioma: Growth, cytology, tumorigenicity and consistent chromosome findings in cell lines from five patients. *Carcinogenesis* **11:** 673.

Popescu, N.C., A.P. Chahinian, and J.A. Dipaolo. 1988. Nonrandom chromosome alterations in human malignant mesothelioma. *Cancer Res.* **48:** 142.

Rappold, G.A., T. Cremer, H.D. Hager, K.E. Davies, C.R. Müller, and T. Yang. 1984. Sex chromosome positions in human interphase nuclei as studied by in situ hybridization with chromosome specific DNA probes. *Hum. Genet.* **67:** 317.

Rey, J.A., M.J. Bello, J.M. De Campos, M.E. Kusak, S. Moreno, and J. Benitez. 1987. Deletion 3p in two lung adenocarcinomas metastatic to the brain. *Cancer Genet. Cytogenet.* **25:** 355.

Sandberg, A.A. 1986. Chromosome changes in bladder cancer: Clinical and other correlations. *Cancer Genet. Cytogenet.* **19:** 163.

Stenman, G., K. Olofsson, T. Månsson, B. Hagmar, and J. Mark. 1986. Chromosomes and chromosomal evolution in human mesotheliomas as reflected in sequential analyses of two cases. *Hereditas* **105:** 233.

Tiainen, M., L. Tammilehto, K. Mattson, and S. Knuutila. 1988. Nonrandom chromosomal abnormalities in malignant pleural mesothelioma. *Cancer Genet. Cytogenet.* **33:** 251.

Tiainen, M., L. Tammilehto, J. Rautonen, T. Tuomi, K. Mattson, and S. Knuutila. 1989. Chromosomal abnormalities and their correlations with asbestos exposure and survival in patients with mesothelioma. *Br. J. Cancer* **60:** 618.

Tuomi, T., M. Segerberg-Konttinen, L. Tammilehto, A. Tossavainen, and E. Vanhala. 1989. Mineral fiber concentration in lung tissue of mesothelioma patients in Finland. *Am. J. Ind. Med.* **16:** 247.

Wessman, M. and S. Knuutila. 1988. A method for the determination of cell morphology, immunologic phenotype and numerical chromosomal abnormalities on the same mitotic or interphase cancer cell. *Genet. Life Sci. Adv.* **7:** 127.

Whang-Peng, J., P.A. Bunn, Jr., C.S. Kao-Shan, E.C. Lee, D.N. Carney, A. Gazdar, and J.D. Minna. 1982. A nonrandom chromosomal abnormality. del3p(14-23), in human small cell lung cancer (SCLC). *Cancer Genet. Cytogenet.* **6:** 119.

Zang, K.D. 1982. Cytological and cytogenetical studies on human meningioma. *Cancer Genet. Cytogenet.* **6:** 249.

Biology of Normal, Malignant, and Oncogene-transfected Human Mesothelial Cells in Culture

T.M. O'Connell[1,3] and J.G. Rheinwald[1,2,3]
[1]Division of Cell Growth and Regulation
Dana-Farber Cancer Institute
Boston, Massachusetts 02115
[2]Department of Cellular and Molecular Physiology
Harvard Medical School
Boston, Massachusetts 02115

INTRODUCTION

The mesothelium is the simple squamous epithelium that lines the pleural, pericardial, and peritoneal cavities and covers the outer surfaces of the lungs, heart, and viscera that are contained within these cavities. It functions as a slippery surface on which the internal organs slide (Cunningham 1926; Andrews and Porter 1973). The mesothelium is unusual among epithelial tissues in that it is derived developmentally from the embryonic mesoderm rather than from the ectoderm or the endoderm. The ability to culture serially pure populations of cells from various human epithelial tissues has advanced research directed at understanding mechanisms of their growth regulation, differentiation, and malignant transformation. The growth factor and nutritional requirements of normal human mesothelial cells for proliferation in culture have been identified previously (Connell and Rheinwald 1983; for review, see Rheinwald 1989). We have used this culture system to elucidate several important growth and differentiation regulatory mechanisms that operate in this cell type and that become altered as a consequence of malignant transformation.

[3]Present address: Biosurface Technology, Inc., One Kendall Square, Cambridge, Massachusetts 02139.

Cellular and Molecular Aspects of Fiber Carcinogenesis
Copyright 1991 Cold Spring Harbor Laboratory Press 0-87969-361-4/91 $1.00 + 00

Initiation of Primary Cultures and Serial Cultivation of Normal Human Mesothelial Cells

The body cavities are normally "potential spaces," containing very little fluid. Patients with metastatic cancer in one of these cavities often accumulate liters of "ascites" fluid (in the peritoneum) or "effusion" fluid (in the pleura or pericardium). It has long been known that normal human mesothelial cells slough off into this fluid (see, e.g., Cunningham 1922; Castor and Naylor 1969; Singh et al. 1978; Domagala and Koss 1979). Our investigations of the mesothelial cell began with the discovery that our attempts at culturing ovarian carcinoma cells from ascites fluid invariably resulted in the selective growth of normal mesothelial cells under our culture conditions (Wu et al. 1982). Soon thereafter, we identified an optimal culture medium for human mesothelial cells, consisting of a 1:1 mixture (v/v) of M199 and either MCDB202 or MCDB105, supplemented with 5–10 ng/ml epidermal growth factor (EGF), 0.4 ug/ml hydrocortisone (HC), and ≥5% bovine serum (Connell and Rheinwald 1983; Rheinwald 1989). In this medium, normal human mesothelial cells grow from very-low-density platings and can be serially passaged with a population-doubling time of ≤24 hours. The growth requirements of human mesothelial cells and their sensitivities to growth inhibitors are very different from those of keratinocytes (i.e., stratified squamous epithelial cells), fibroblasts, and large-vessel endothelial cells (Table 1).

Mesothelial cells have a very distinctive morphology in culture. They do not form closely adherent colonies as do other epithelial cell types. In their optimal growth medium, they adopt a stubby, somewhat fibroblastoid morphology and grow in a dispersed fashion. However, mesothelial cells are not as long and spindly as human fibroblasts. They form a broad, ruffled plasma membrane along one side, and they migrate laterally. Under optimal growth conditions, they mimic fibroblasts by continuing to divide after reaching a confluent monolayer, ultimately forming a multilayer of elongated cells at saturation densities of up to 2×10^5 cells/cm^2. If EGF is withdrawn from preconfluent cultures, however, mesothelial cells flatten, slow their growth to a doubling time of ≥80 hours,

TABLE 1 MITOGEN REQUIREMENTS AND INHIBITOR SENSITIVITIES OF NORMAL HUMAN MESOTHELIAL CELLS AND OTHER CELL TYPES

Factor[a]	Cell type[b]			
	mesothelial	keratinocyte	fibroblast	endothelial
EGF	R	R	s	–
FGF	R	s	s	R
HC	R	R	–	s
High [Ade]	I	S	I	I
Insulin	s	S	s	s
CT	–	S	I	–
Feeders	–	R	–	–
Serum	R	–	R	R
Complex medium	R	–	s	s
TGF-β	–	I	–	–
TPA	–	I	–	–

[a]Abbreviations and explanations: (EGF) epidermal growth factor; (FGF) fibroblast growth factor; (HC) hydrocortisone; (high [Ade]) 1.8×10^{-4} M; (CT) cholera toxin; (feeders) 3T3 fibroblast feeder layer; (serum) nondialyzable serum factors; (complex medium) grows in M199/MCDB105 but not in DME/F12; (TGF-β) transforming growth factor-β; (TPA) 12-0-tetradecanoylphorbol-13-acetate.
[b](R) Required; (S) strongly stimulatory; (s) weakly stimulatory; (I) inhibitory; (–) little or no effect.

and form an epithelioid monolayer at a saturation density of approximately 3×10^4 cells/cm^2, resembling their normal in vivo histology (Connell and Rheinwald 1983). As is true for human cells of all types, mesothelial cells remain diploid and retain their morphological and growth factor requirement characteristics during a finite replicative life span in culture, which for mesothelial cells obtained from adults is 40–50 cell generations.

Plasminogen Activator Inhibitor Production by Cultured Mesothelial Cells

Human mesothelial cells in culture synthesize and secrete very large amounts of a 46-kD glycoprotein that we originally named "mesosecrin" (Rheinwald et al. 1987). Our attempts to determine its sequence and function (Cicila et al. 1989) led us to the discovery that mesosecrin is actually plasminogen activator inhibitor type-1 (PAI-1) (Andreasen et al. 1986; Ginsburg et al. 1986; Ny et al. 1986; Pannekoek et al. 1986; Wun and Kretzmer 1987). Human mesothelial, endothelial, and type II kidney epithelial cells (one of the two cell types that proliferate in culture from explanted human kidney cortex [Rheinwald and O'Connell 1985]) devote approximately 5% of their total protein synthesis in culture to PAI-1, whereas keratinocytes, urothelial cells, conjunctival epithelial cells, and mammary epithelial cells do not synthesize detectable amounts of this protein under normal culture conditions. Indirect immuno-fluorescence reveals that mesothelial cells deposit PAI-1 beneath themselves as a fine coating on the culture sub-stratum, and from there it is subsequently released into the medium (Rheinwald et al. 1987).

PAI-1 promotes fibrin clot stability (for review, see Spreng-ers and Kluft 1987) and is believed to play an important role in modulating cell migration, tissue destruction and remodeling, and neoplastic and non-neoplastic invasiveness (for review, see Dano et al. 1985). It is surprising that mesothelial cells and endothelial cells synthesize such large amounts of PAI-1 in culture since, under normal circumstances in vivo, these cell types function to *prevent* clot formation and to *promote* fibrinolysis. One explanation is that, when mesothelial and endothelial cells are induced to adhere to plastic and divide in culture, they adopt a state similar to that of wound healing in vivo. Under these circumstances, temporary inhibition of fibrin degradation would be a useful function. Polarized secretion of PAI-1 through the basal surface of the cell with deposition onto the substratum could also serve to maintain the integrity of the basement membrane in vivo and thereby help stabilize the fragile, simple squamous cell sheet. On the other hand, abnormal apical or nonpolarized secretion of PAI-1 by meso-thelial cells could be the cause of the pathological deposition of fibrin and consequent adhesions that frequently occur in in-fection and inflammation of the pleura and pericardial cavities.

Growth Regulation and Reversible Dedifferentiation of Cultured Human Mesothelial Cells

In vivo, mesothelial cells exist in a nondividing state and have a high content of keratin-type intermediate filaments and a low but detectable content of vimentin intermediate filaments (Franke et al. 1978; Schlegel et al. 1980; Corson and Pinkus 1982; LaRocca and Rheinwald 1984). In the course of our investigation of the EGF-dependent growth of mesothelial cells in culture, we discovered one of their interesting and unique properties; the reversible loss of keratin by cells during rapid growth (Connell and Rheinwald 1983). Mesothelial cells synthesize a set of four keratin subunit proteins known as the "simple epithelial keratins" (Moll et al. 1982) that we originally called "mesothelial keratins" (Wu et al. 1982): K7, K8, K18, K19 ($\sim M_r$ 55,000, 52,000, 44,000, and 40,000, respectively). Within several days of being placed in primary culture in their optimal growth medium, the cells assume their characteristic in vitro morphology, described above. This morphologic conversion from that of the quiescent in vivo state to that of the rapidly growing in vitro state is accompanied by a decrease in keratin synthesis and content, an increase in vimentin synthesis and content (Connell and Rheinwald 1983), and the synthesis and secretion of large amounts of fibronectin (Rheinwald et al. 1987). Keratin synthesis and content returns to high levels whenever EGF is removed from the medium and cell growth slows, and they assume their flattened epithelioid morphology. The turnover rate of keratins is very slow and is the same for growing and quiescent cells. Thus, differences in keratin content are determined completely by changes in the rate of keratin synthesis and whether dilution of previously accumulated keratins occurs as a consequence of cell division (Connell and Rheinwald 1983). Rapidly growing mesothelial cells have much less keratin mRNA than do cells that are quiescent in the absence of EGF. Thus, changes in the rate of keratin synthesis are regulated at the level of mRNA (Rheinwald et al. 1984).

This reversible dedifferentiation that is modulated by extrinsic signals is very different from the continual synthesis of keratins by keratinocytes during serial culture and the irreversible loss of proliferation potential by keratinocytes before they can complete their differentiation program. Interestingly, another mesoderm-derived cell type, the type II kidney epithelial cell, closely resembles the mesothelial cell with respect to characteristics of growth regulation and intermediate filament

protein expression in culture (Rheinwald et al. 1984; Rheinwald and O'Connell 1985). Both convert during embryogenesis
from nonepithelioid progenitor cells dispersed in a connective
tissue-like extracellular matrix to polarized epithelial cells pos-
sessing a distinctive apical surface and resting on a basement
membrane. Perhaps these cell types retain the ability to regulate intermediate filament content and fibronectin production
to facilitate the performance of alternate functions of growth/
wound repair and squamous epithelium formation. This would
seem especially beneficial to the fragile mesothelium, which is
susceptible to damage by abrasion and inflammation.

The remarkable capacity of normal mesothelial cells to
dedifferentiate reversibly or to "transdifferentiate" to a fibroblastoid phenotype explains the striking histologic heterogeneity of mesotheliomas, many of which contain both epithelioid
and fibroblastoid regions (see Klemperer and Rabin 1931;
Stout and Murray 1942; Corson and Pinkus 1982). Because of
their histopathologic appearance, mesotheliomas were once
regarded as fibrosarcomas. However, mesothelioma cells in
tumors merely exhibit the phenotypic range that is exhibited
by normal mesothelial cells in culture. This helps to explain
why some, but not all, of the fibroblastoid cells within
mesotheliomas are stained by anti-keratin antibodies (Schlegel
et al. 1980). It seems that, during malignant transformation,
mesothelial cells lose their dependence on external mitogens,
convert from a quiescent to a growing state, and therefore also
begin to express a fibroblast-like differentiation program.

Mesothelioma-derived Cell Lines and Oncogene-transfected
Mesothelial Cells: Mitogen Independence and
Growth Factor Secretion

Many cell lines derived from human malignant mesothelioma
exhibit mitogen-independent growth in culture (A.J. Terpstra
and J.G. Rheinwald, unpubl.). We found that the mesothelioma line JMN1B (a subline that we isolated from the JMN line
of Behbehani et al. [1982]) grows optimally without the addition of EGF to the culture medium and secretes a mitogen
(transformed mesothelial growth factor [TMGF]) that can
satisfy the EGF requirement of normal human mesothelial

cells. Our discovery of these interesting characteristics of JMN1B cells led us to analyze the phenotypic changes that result from the introduction of specific oncogenes into normal diploid mesothelial cells.

Human mesothelial cells are efficient recipients of foreign DNA using calcium-phosphate, lipid-vesicle, and retrovirus-mediated transfection. When a mutationally activated Ha-*ras* gene (Tubo and Rheinwald 1987) or the gene encoding the SV40 large T antigen (SVLT) (G.T. Cicila and J.G. Rheinwald, unpubl.) are introduced into normal mesothelial cells, the resulting transfectants exhibit morphologic alterations, disorganized growth patterns, and mitogen-independent growth. The *ras* transfectants are independent of EGF for rapid growth, but they are not immortal nor do they form tumors in athymic *nude* mice. The SVLT transfectants are EGF- and hydrocortizone (HC)-independent and also exhibit a reduced requirement for serum. Some SVLT transfectants escape senescence and become replicatively immortal. They are not, however, tumorigenic in *nude* mice. An examination of the conditioned medium from these experimentally transfected cells revealed the presence of a mitogen with the same biological activity as that which is secreted by the JMN1B line.

Normal human mesothelial cells can be induced in culture to synthesize and secrete a number of lymphokines, including granulocyte-colony-stimulating factor (G-CSF), granulocyte-macrophage-colony-stimulating factor (GM-CSF), macrophage-colony-stimulating factor (M-CSF), and interleukin-1β (IL-1β), by exposure to inflammatory mediators such as bacterial endotoxin (lipopolysaccharide [LPS]) or tumor necrosis factor (TNF) (Demetri et al. 1989). EGF and TNF act synergistically to induce maximal levels of G-CSF and GM-CSF transcripts. The presence of either EGF, TNF, or LPS alone induces mesothelial cells to synthesize increased levels of IL-1β mRNA. Glucocorticoids oppose the induction of the IL-1β message by EGF or TNF. Interestingly, the EGF-independent mesothelioma line JMN1B and *ras* oncogene-transfected cells exhibit autonomous expression of G-CSF, GM-CSF, M-CSF, IL-1β, and IL-6 mRNA (Demetri et al. 1989, 1990). Thus, transformation of the mesothelial cell is accompanied by the unregulated expression of a large number of growth factors, one of which (TMGF) is an autocrine mitogen for mesothelial cells. Our experiments have demonstrated that neither G-CSF, M-CSF, nor GM-CSF are mitogenic to mesothelial cells and that IL-1β is only a very weak mesothelial mitogen; thus, TMGF is different from any of these factors.

We are currently in the process of characterizing TMGF (B.W. Zenzie et al., in prep.). Antibody neutralization and receptor-blocking experiments show that TMGF is not EGF or transforming growth factor-α (TGF-α) nor any other factor that acts via the EGF receptor. Pure acidic and basic FGF have become available since our earlier analyses of mesothelial cell mitogenic requirements (Connell and Rheinwald 1983; La-Rocca and Rheinwald 1985; Tubo and Rheinwald 1987), and we have found that these factors can satisfy the "EGF requirement" of normal mesothelial cells. However, PDGF, TGF-β, and insulin-like growth factor cannot. TMGF shares some properties with basic FGF in that both induce neurite extension of PC-12 cells and the mitogenic activities of both are inhibited by heparin. However, radioimmunoassay using an antiserum specific for basic FGF has revealed that TMGF is not basic FGF. We have also found that TMGF is nonmitogenic to large-vessel endothelial cells, which also clearly proves the non-identity of TMGF and basic FGF. Biogel P100 gel filtration chromatography of JMNIB-conditioned medium fractionates most of the TMGF activity as a large protein or complex (≥66 kD), but some mitogenically active fractions elute with an apparent molecular mass of 16–20 kD. At the time of this writing, we are working to characterize TMGF more precisely.

Normal human mesothelial cells in culture represent an important experimental system for studying epithelial cell biology and oncogenesis. As described above, the growth factor requirements and differentiation of this interesting and unusual cell type have been characterized in detail. Mesothelial cells are also very amenable to genetic manipulation, thus facilitating molecular studies of the aberrations in cell regulation exhibited by mesothelioma cells. Perhaps the most important change associated with mesothelial cell transformation is the expression of a novel autocrine growth factor. This mitogen has the ability to activate growth and dedifferentiation in the normally quiescent epithelioid mesothelium. Thus, its characterization and the pattern of its expression during oncogenesis merit further research.

ACKNOWLEDGMENTS

We thank all of the former members of our laboratory whose research results are reviewed in this publication, particularly Anita Terpstra, George Cicila, and Beatrice Zenzie, whose unpublished results we have mentioned. Philip Connell, Damon Graff, and Christy Stotler provided excellent technical assistance. Susan Sullivan skillfully prepared the manuscript. These investigations were supported by grants to J.G.R. from The National Institute on Aging, The National Foundation for Cancer Research, the National Cancer Institute, and by an American Cancer Society Faculty Research Award to J.G.R.

REFERENCES

Andreasen, P.A., A. Riccio, K.G. Welinder, R. Douglas, R. Sartorio, L.S. Nielsen, C. Oppenheimer, F. Blasi, and K. Dano. 1986. Plasminogen activator inhibitor type-1: Reactive center and aminoterminal heterogeneity determined by protein and cDNA sequencing. *FEBS Lett.* **209:** 213.

Andrews, P.M. and K.R. Porter. 1973. The ultra-structural, morphology and possible functional significance of mesothelial microvilli. *Anat. Rec.* **177:** 409.

Behbehani, A.M., W.J. Hunter, A.L. Chapman, and F. Lin. 1982. Studies of a human mesothelioma. *Hum. Pathol.* **13:** 862.

Castor, C.W. and B. Naylor. 1969. Characteristics of normal and malignant human mesothelial cells studied *in vitro*. *Lab Invest.* **20:** 437.

Cicila, G.T., T.M. O'Connell, W.C. Hahn, and J.G. Rheinwald. 1989. Cloned cDNA sequences for the human mesothelial protein "mesosecrin" discloses its identity as a plasminogen activator inhibitor (PAI-1) and a recent evolutionary change in transcript processing. *J. Cell Sci.* **94:** 1.

Connell, N.D. and J.G. Rheinwald. 1983. Regulation of the cytoskeleton in mesothelial cells: Reversible loss of keratin and increase in vimentin during rapid growth in culture. *Cell* **34:** 245.

Corson, J.M. and G.S. Pinkus. 1982. Mesothelioma: Profile of keratin proteins and carcinoembryonic antigen. An immunoperoxidase study of 20 cases and comparison with pulmonary adenocarcinomas. *Am. J. Pathol.* **108:** 80.

Cunningham, R.S. 1922. On the origin of the free cells of serous exudates. *Am. J. Physiol.* **59:** 1.

———. 1926. The physiology of the serous membranes. *Physiol. Rev.* **6:** 242.

Dano, K., P.A. Andreasen, J. Grondahl-Hansen, P. Kristensen, L.S. Nielsen, and L. Skriver. 1985. Plasminogen activators, tissue degradation, and cancer. *Adv. Cancer Res.* **44:** 139.

Demetri, G.D., B.W. Zenzie, J.G. Rheinwald, and J.D. Griffin. 1989. Expression of colony-stimulating factor genes by normal human mesothelial cells and human malignant mesothelioma cell lines *in vitro. Blood* **74:** 940.

Demetri, G.D., T.J. Ernst, E.S. Pratt, B.W. Zenzie, J.G. Rheinwald, and J.D. Griffin. 1990. Expression of *ras* oncogenes in cultured human cells alters the transcriptional and postranscriptional regulation of cytokine genes. *J. Clin. Invest.* **86:** 1261.

Domagala, W. and L.G. Koss. 1979. Surface configuration of mesothelial cells in effusions. *Virchows Arch. B Cell Pathol.* **30:** 231.

Franke, W.W., E. Schmid, M. Osborn, and K. Weber. 1978. Different intermediate-sized filaments distinguished by immunofluorescence microscopy. *Proc. Natl. Acad. Sci.* **75:** 5034.

Ginsburg, D., R. Zeheb, A.Y. Yang, U.M. Rafferty, P.A. Andreasen, L. Nielsen, K. Dano, R.V. Lebo, and T.D. Gelehrter. 1986. cDNA cloning of human plasminogen activator-inhibitor from endothelial cells. *J. Clin. Invest.* **78:** 1673.

Klemperer, P. and C.B. Rabin. 1931. Primary neoplasms of the pleura. *Arch. Pathol.* **11:** 385.

LaRocca, P.J. and J.G. Rheinwald. 1984. Coexpression of simple epithelial keratins and vimentin by human mesothelium and mesothelioma *in vivo* and in culture. *Cancer Res.* **44:** 2991.

———. 1985. Anchorage-independent growth of normal human mesothelial cells: A sensitive bioassay for EGF which discloses the absence of this factor in fetal calf serum. *In Vitro* **21:** 67.

Moll, R., W.W. Franke, D.L. Schiller, B. Geiger, and R. Krepler. 1982. The catalog of human cytokeratins: Patterns of expression in normal epithelia, tumors and cultured cells. *Cell* **31:** 11.

Ny, T., M. Sawdey, D. Lawrence, J.L. Millan, and D.J. Loskutoff. 1986. Cloning and sequence of a cDNA coding for the human B-migrating endothelial cell-type plasminogen activator inhibitor. *Proc. Natl. Acad. Sci.* **83:** 6776.

Pannekoek, H., H. Veerman, H. Lambers, P. Diergaarde, C.L. Verweij, A.-J. van Zonneveld, and J.A. Mourik. 1986. Endothelial plasminogen activator inhibitor (PAI): A new member of the serpine gene family. *EMBO J.* **5:** 2539.

Rheinwald, J.G. 1989. Methods for clonal growth and serial cultivation of normal epidermal keroatinocytes and mesothelial cells. In *Cell growth and division: A practical approach* (ed. R. Baserga), p. 81. IRL Press, Oxford, England.

Rheinwald, J.G. and T.M. O'Connell. 1985. Intermediate filament proteins as distinguishing markers of cell type and differentiated state in cultured human urinary tract epithelia. *Ann. N.Y. Acad. Sci.* **455**: 259.

Rheinwald, J.G., J.L. Jorgensen, W.C. Hahn, A.J. Terpstra, T.M. O'Connell, and K.K. Plummer. 1987. Mesosecrin: A secreted glycoprotein produced in abundance by human mesothelial, endothelial, and kidney epithelial cells in culture. *J. Cell Biol.* **104**: 263.

Rheinwald, J.G., T.M. O'Connell, N.D. Connell, S.M. Rybak, B.L. Allen-Hoffmann, P.J. LaRocca, Y.-J. Wu, and S.M. Rehwoldt. 1984. Expression of specific keratin subsets and vimentin in normal human epithelial cells: A function of cell type and conditions of growth during serial culture. *Cancer Cells* **1**: 217.

Schlegel, R., S. Banks-Schlegel, J.A. McLeod, and G.S. Pinkus. 1980. Immunoperoxidase localization of keratin in human neoplasms. *Am. J. Pathol.* **101**: 41.

Singh, G., A. Dekker, and C.T. Ladoulis. 1978. Tissue culture of cells in serous effusions: Evaluation as an adjunct to cytology. *Acta Cytol.* **22**: 487.

Stout, A.P. and M.R. Murray. 1942. Localized pleural mesothelioma. *Arch. Pathol.* **34**: 951.

Sprengers, E.D. and C. Kluft. 1987. Plasminogen activator inhibitors. *Blood* **69**: 381.

Tubo, R.A. and J.G. Rheinwald. 1987. Normal human mesothelial cells and fibroblasts transfected with the EJ *ras* oncogene become EGF-independent, but are not malignantly transformed. *Oncogene Res.* **1**: 407.

Wu, Y.-J., L.M. Parker, N.E. Binder, M.A. Beckett, J.H. Sinard, C.T. Griffiths, and J.G. Rheinwald. 1982. The mesothelial keratins: A new family of cytoskeletal proteins identified in cultured mesothelial cells and non-keratinizing epithelia. *Cell* **31**: 693.

Wun, T.-C. and K.K. Kretzmer. 1987. cDNA cloning and expression in *E. coli* of a plasminogen activator inhibitor (PAI) related to a PAI produced by Hep G2 hepatoma cell. *FEBS Lett.* **210**: 11.

Oncogenes and Signal Transduction in Malignancy

C.J. Molloy,[1] T.P. Fleming, D.P. Bottaro, A. Cuadrado, M.J. Pangelinan, and S.A. Aaronson

Laboratory of Cellular and Molecular Biology, National Cancer Institute
Bethesda, Maryland 20892

INTRODUCTION

There is increasing evidence that oncogenes encoding proteins that are homologous to either growth factors or growth factor receptors play an important role in the development of certain malignancies. For example, the v-*sis* oncogene product of the simian sarcoma virus is derived from the gene encoding the B-chain of the platelet-derived growth factor (PDGF) (Doolittle et al. 1983; Waterfield et al. 1983). In addition, v-*erbB* and v-*fms* are derived from the genes encoding the epidermal growth factor (Downward et al. 1984) and colony-stimulating factor-1 (Sherr et al. 1985) receptors, respectively. A further linkage between growth control and oncogenes is that the common tyrosine kinase activity associated with many activated growth factor receptors is shared with several viral oncogene products (Hunter and Cooper 1985). These findings have spirited the investigation of growth factor signaling pathways involving tyrosine kinases in an attempt to understand the biochemical mechanisms involved in normal growth and malignancy.

Possible Role of PDGF Gene Expression in Malignancy, Including Mesothelioma

The introduction of an expression vector containing the normal human *sis*/PDGF-BB homodimer-coding sequence into

---

[1]Present address: Department of Cardiovascular Biochemistry, Bristol-Meyers Squibb Pharmaceutical Research Institute, Princeton, New Jersey 08543.

Cellular and Molecular Aspects of Fiber Carcinogenesis
Copyright 1991 Cold Spring Harbor Laboratory Press 0-87969-361-4/91 $1.00 + 00 **67**

continuous mouse fibroblast lines in culture can confer the malignant phenotype (Gazit et al. 1984). These findings have implied that the induction of growth factor production in cells expressing the appropriate receptor(s) can be an important step in the development of malignancy, allowing cells to by-pass the need for exogenously controlled proliferation signals (for review, see Sporn and Roberts 1985). Recently, several studies have indicated that the increased expression of genes encoding PDGF is a common occurrence in malignant meso-thelioma. Gerwin et al. (1987) have detected an increase in mRNA for both PDGF-A and/or PDGF-B chains in several human mesothelioma cell lines. Similarly, Versnel et al. (1988) have shown that human mesothelioma cell lines derived from primary and metastatic sites strongly overexpressed the c-*sis* (PDGF-B chain) gene when compared with normal mesothelial cells. Thus, elucidation of the exact mechanisms involved in cell transformation by overexpression of genes encoding the PDGF growth factor family may be critical in development of new treatments for this invariably fatal disease.

Site of PDGF Receptor Activation and Functional Coupling with Mitogenic Signaling Pathways in Fibroblasts Transformed by the sis Oncogene

Efforts to establish whether autocrine growth stimulation can be blocked by specific surface receptor antagonists have in-tensified. Previous efforts to localize the site of v-*sis* action have led to conflicting findings and conclusions. Antibody to PDGF has been reported to inhibit growth of v-*sis* transfor-mants to varying extents, which is consistent with at least some surface component to activity of the v-*sis* product (Hu-ang et al. 1984; Johnsson et al. 1985). Moreover, Hannink and Donoghue (1988) reported that v-*sis* products that failed to achieve a cell-surface site lacked transforming activity. In con-trast, other investigators have reported evidence that internal forms of the PDGF receptor (PDGFR) are tyrosine phosphory-lated and exhibit greatly increased turnover in the absence of detectable mature PDGFR species (Huang and Huang 1988; Keating and Williams 1988). This has led to a so-called "inter-nal autocrine" model, implying that receptor activation and functional coupling with mitogenic pathways occurs entirely within the cell.

Clinical intervention in malignancies involving activated growth factor receptors may be more readily achieved if functional activation of the receptor occurs at the cell surface. Although not generally expressed by the same cells, growth factors and their receptors are often processed through the same secretory pathway (Farquhar 1985; Robbins et al. 1985). Moreover, in the case of the v-*sis*/PDGF-B product, immature dimeric forms that are present only within the cell have been shown to have mitogenic potential (Leal et al. 1985). Efforts to localize the critical site(s) for functional interaction of the v-*sis*-encoded protein with PDGFRs have resulted in contradictory conclusions. Current models predict either that mitogenically active v-*sis* gene products bind and activate PDGFRs during processing within the cell or that functional interaction occurs only after these molecules achieve a cell-surface location. Our recent studies have attempted to establish the specific sites of receptor activation and functional coupling with mitogenic signal-transduction pathways. These findings have general implications concerning localization within the cell of critical targets of growth-factor-receptor action and approaches toward intervention with autocrine-associated malignancies (Fleming et al. 1989).

Exogenously Added PDGF Transiently Mimics the v-sis-*transformed Phenotype in Fibroblasts*

Reproduction of the v-*sis*-transformed phenotype could be achieved by the exogenous stimulation of nontransformed NIH-3T3 cells with purified PDGF-BB homodimer. When cells were maintained in a medium that was supplemented daily with 3 ng/ml PDGF-BB, their morphology was indistinguishable from that of v-*sis* transformants (Fig. 1A–C). Moreover, such cells formed colonies in soft agar at an efficiency comparable with that of v-*sis* transformants (Fig. 1D–F). Thus, chronic activation of PDGFRs at the cell surface may be sufficient for v-*sis* transformation.

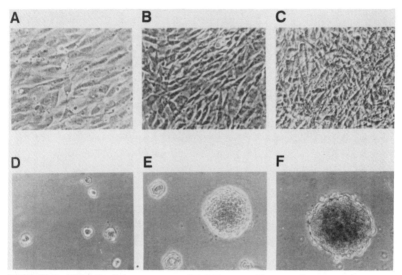

FIGURE 1 Effect of exogenous PDGF on cell-growth properties. NIH-3T3 cells (*A, D*) or v-*sis*-transformed NIH-3T3 cells (*B, E*) were grown in Dulbecco's modified Eagle's medium containing 10% calf serum. Some NIH-3T3 cell cultures (*C, F*) were supplemented daily with 3 ng of PDGF-BB. Appearance of cells after 7 days in liquid control (*A, B, C*) or semisolid 0.4% agar suspension (*D, E, F*). Magnification, 135x.

Partial Growth Inhibition by a PDGF Neutralizing Antibody Establishes a Surface Component to Activity of the v-sis Protein

To explore the degree to which transforming activity of the v-*sis* gene product might be susceptible to intervention at the cell surface, a neutralizing PDGF antibody was used in conjunction with cell-culture conditions in which DNA synthesis by v-*sis*-transformed cells was completely dependent on v-*sis* expression (Fleming et al. 1989). Thus, in a chemically defined medium in which control NIH-3T3 cells failed to grow unless supplemented with PDGF-BB, v-*sis* transformants proliferated without added PDGF-BB. Under these conditions, 50 µg/ml PDGF neutralizing antibody completely inhibited DNA synthesis by NIH-3T3 cells exposed to PDGF-BB (Fig. 2) but had no effect on *erbB2*-transformed cells even at an antibody concentration of 500 µg/ml. The same antibody was able to inhibit thymidine incorporation by v-*sis*-transformed cells by

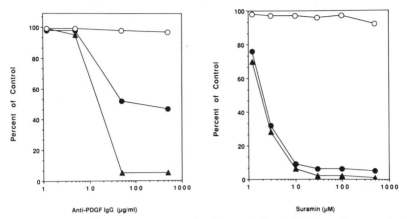

FIGURE 2 (*Left*) Anti-PDGF antibody partially inhibits mitogenesis in v-*sis*-transformed cells. DNA synthesis was measured after 24 hr exposure to varying anti-PDGF immunoglobulin G (IgG) concentrations. Results were normalized to those obtained with untreated cultures and represent mean values of at least triplicate determinations. Control NIH-3T3 cells were plated in chemically defined medium containing 3 ng/ml PDGF-BB (closed triangles); v-*sis* (closed circles), and *erbB2* (open circles) transformants were plated in medium lacking PDGF-BB. (*Right*) Effect of suramin on DNA synthesis of PDGF-BB-stimulated control or v-*sis*-transformed NIH-3T3 cells. DNA synthesis was measured following a 24-hr exposure to varying suramin concentrations. Results were normalized to those obtained with untreated cultures and represent mean values of at least triplicate determinations. Control NIH-3T3 cells were plated on chemically defined medium containing 3 ng/ml of PDGF-BB (closed triangles), v-*sis* (closed circles), and *erbB2* (open circles) transformants were plated in medium lacking PDGF-BB.

approximately 50% (Fig. 2). These data indicate that the functional activity of the v-*sis* product was susceptible at least in part to intervention at the cell surface.

Complete Inhibition of v-sis Transformation by Suramin Provides a Biochemical Tool in Mechanistic Studies

Suramin is an anionic naphthalene sulfonic acid derivative that has been used for over 50 years in the pharmacological therapy of trypanosomiasis (for review, see LaRocca et al. 1990). This drug has also been reported to inhibit PDGF mitogenic activity and to induce transient reversion of the v-*sis*-

transformed phenotype (Betsholtz et al. 1986; Keating and Williams 1988). However, evidence that suramin may act within the cell as well as externally has led to controversy concerning its mechanism of action. In our studies, we investigated the ability of suramin to inhibit v-sis-directed cell proliferation using the chemically defined system described above. As shown in Figure 2, suramin induced a dose-dependent inhibition of DNA synthesis in v-sis-transformed cells and in cells stimulated by exogenous PDGF-BB. As a control, suramin failed to inhibit DNA synthesis by erbB2-transformed cells under the same conditions. The inhibitory effect of suramin on exogenously added PDGF or v-sis-directed proliferation was also apparent in a time course study, where inhibition in each case was greater than 95% over 72 hours. All of these findings demonstrated that suramin was a more potent inhibitor than PDGF antibody of v-sis-directed growth and thus potentially provided a means to assess the key biochemical events involved in v-sis transformation.

Functional Coupling of Activated PDGF Receptors with Intracellular Mitogenic Signaling Pathways is Confined to the Cell Surface in v-sis Transformation

Recent investigations have demonstrated that two distinct genes encode PDGFRs (Matsui et al. 1989) and that both of these genes are expressed in fibroblasts. The α-PDGFR gene product can be activated, as evidenced by its ability to undergo protein tyrosine autophosphorylation, in response to all three PDGF isoforms including AA, AB, and BB (Matsui et al. 1989). In contrast, the PDGFR-β gene product does not appear to interact with the AA isoform (for review, see Heldin and Westermark 1989). To investigate PDGFR activation in v-sis-transformed cells, we used antipeptide antibodies specific for each receptor (Matsui et al. 1989). Cell lysates were first specifically enriched for the respective receptors by immunoprecipitation, which was then followed by immunoblot analysis using an affinity-purified anti-phosphotyrosine-antiserum (Fleming et al. 1989). In v-sis-transformed NIH-3T3 cells, we observed tyrosine phosphorylated cell-surface α and β receptors at levels approximating those of NIH-3T3 cells exposed for

Anti-P-Tyr

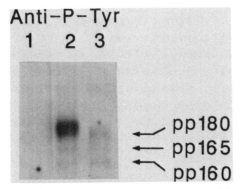

FIGURE 3 Comparison of suramin effects on tyrosine-phosphorylated mature and immature type α- and β-PDGF receptor species. Lysates of untreated NIH-3T3 (lane *1*), untreated v-*sis*-transformed NIH-3T3 (lane *2*), or v-*sis*-transformed NIH-3T3 cells exposed to 100 μM suramin for 24 hr (lane *3*) were immunoprecipitated with anti-phosphotyrosine serum and subjected to SDS polyacrylamide gel electrophoresis. (pp180) Mature forms of α- and β-PDGFRs; (pp165) intracellular form of the β-PDGFR; (pp160) intracellular form of the α-PDGFR.

18 hours to PDGF-BB. These receptors migrate as 180-kD proteins in SDS-polyacrylamide gels (Fig. 3, lane 2). Of note, the v-*sis*-transformed cells also contained detectable tyrosine-phosphorylated immature forms of both receptors that consist of an incompletely glycosylated lower-molecular-weight species of the respective receptors (α-type receptor, 160 kD; β-type receptor, 165 kD; see Keating and Williams 1988; Matsui et al. 1989). Thus, in v-*sis*-transformed fibroblasts, both immature and surface forms of both PDGFRs are activated.

To establish the site at which suramin blocked the function of the v-*sis* product, v-*sis*-transformed cells were first exposed to suramin (100 μM) for 24 hours, and then the status of PDGFR activation was analyzed. Suramin treatment led to a marked diminution in the level of tyrosine phosphorylation of the cell-surface PDGFRs but had no effect on the level of tyrosine phosphorylation of the immature, intracellular α- or PDGFR-β species (Fig. 3, lane 3). Furthermore, we also observed an increase in the actual levels of fully mature, surface-localized PDGFR-α and PDGFR-β indicating receptor "up-regulation" in the presence of suramin (Fleming et al. 1989). Taken together, these results support a model in which the v-sis-encoded mitogen binds and activates PDGFRs at some internal cellular sites (e.g., golgi) but in which the activated receptors must then achieve a cell-surface location to couple functionally with intracellular mitogenic signaling pathways.

It should be noted that our findings do not exclude the possibility that some growth-factor-receptor interactions are first initiated at or "below" the cell surface. Both PDGF antibody and suramin were able to block exogenous PDGF stimulation effectively. Yet, we observed only partial inhibition of v-sis-directed growth by the PDGF neutralizing antibody. If antibody only inhibits de novo ligand binding to receptors, the partial resistance of v-sis-directed proliferation likely reflects antibody-inaccessible ligand already bound to PDGFRs prior to their reaching the cell surface. The total inhibition of v-sis-directed growth induced by suramin suggests that this agent is also able to strip ligands already bound to receptors and to down-regulate enzymatic activity of internally activated receptors as they reach the cell surface.

The evidence that the functional activation of PDGFRs in v-sis transformation requires their cell-surface localization strongly suggests that critical targets of receptor action may be specifically located at or near the inner surface of the cell membrane. If so, surface-acting molecules, which can interfere with ligand-receptor interactions, may have potential applicability in the clinical treatments of autocrine-associated malignancies and other chronic diseases involving autocrine growth stimulation.

Cellular Targets of the Activated PDGFR Tyrosine Kinases

Activation of the intrinsic tyrosine kinase activity of growth-factor receptors resulting in the phosphorylation of important target proteins has been postulated to be a critical event in subsequent mitogenic signal transduction (Hunter and Cooper 1985; Ullrich and Schlessinger 1990). Recent studies of PDGF- and EGF-stimulated cells have identified several putative substrates that may be involved in mitogenic signaling. These include such molecules as phospholipase C-γ (Wahl et al. 1989), phosphatidylinositol kinase (Kaplan et al. 1987), and the c-*raf* protein (Morrison et al. 1989). In general, tyrosine phosphorylation of these proteins has been shown to activate their inherent enzymatic activities, leading to a complex cascade of additional intracellular reactions presumably resulting in altered transcription and translation of growth-related genes.

Functional *ras* proteins have also been implicated in the signal-transduction pathway used by certain growth factors, including PDGF (Mulcahy et al. 1985). These proteins, derived from the family of *ras* genes, are guanine-nucleotide-binding molecules that are commonly activated in human malignancies. Transforming *ras* proteins are potently mitogenic when microinjected into quiescent fibroblasts, yet the function of the endogenous *ras* p21 proteins in normal mitogenic signal transduction remains to be elucidated. It is well established that the GTP-bound forms of *ras* p21 proteins are active and the GDP-bound forms are inactive. Recently, a cytosolic GTPase-activating protein (GAP), of approximately 125 kD, has been shown to catalyze in vivo the conversion of p21 GTP to p21 GDP so that this recycling proceeds at a rate greater than 100-fold in excess of the intrinsic p21 hydrolytic rate (Trahey and McCormick 1987). GAP has no effect on oncogenic *ras* p21 proteins, allowing them to remain in their active GTP-bound states. Since GAP contains sequences similar to certain cytoplasmic tyrosine kinases and tyrosine kinase substrates (Trahey et al. 1988; Vogel et al. 1988), it provided a logical candidate for a substrate of activated tyrosine kinases in intact cells.

Rapid Induction of GAP Tyrosine Phosphorylation in Intact Fibroblasts by PDGF

Confluent NIH-3T3 cells were rendered quiescent by overnight incubation in serum-free medium, and then they were exposed to saturating concentrations of PDGF-BB homodimer for various times. Cell lysates were analyzed using either affinity-purified anti-phosphotyrosine antiserum or anti-GAP peptide

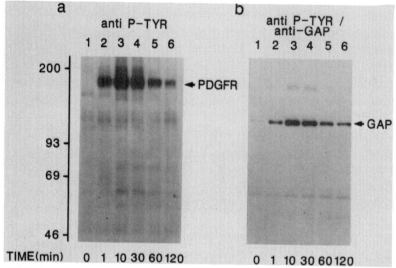

FIGURE 4 Time course of anti-phosphotyrosine recovery of GAP following PDGF-BB stimulation. (*a*) Anti-phosphotyrosine immunoblot analysis of whole-cell lysates from unstimulated cells (lane *1*) and cells stimulated by PDGF-BB for the indicated time (lanes *2–6*). (Arrow) The autophosphorylation of PDGFRs. (*b*) Anti-GAP immunoblot analysis of monoclonal anti-phosphotyrosine immunoprecipitates from cells that are either unstimulated (lane *1*) or stimulated with PDGF-BB for the indicated times (lanes *2–6*). (Arrow) The immunoreactive GAP protein recovered by anti-phosphotyrosine antiserum after PDGF-BB stimulation.

serum in both immunoblotting and immunoprecipitation experiments (Molloy et al. 1989). When quiescent or PDGF-BB-homodimer-treated cells were first immunoprecipitated with anti-phosphotyrosine antiserum and then analyzed by immunoblotting with anti-GAP antiserum, tyrosine phosphorylated GAP was only found in PDGF-BB-stimulated cells (Fig. 4). The data in Figure 4 show that PDGF-BB induced rapid PDGFR autophosphorylation, which increased over the first 10 minutes and then gradually decreased. Similarly, increased anti-phosphotyrosine recovery of GAP could be detected within 1 minute of PDGF addition, was maximal by about 10 minutes, and persisted for at least 2 hours (Fig. 4b). In other experiments, we have detected increased levels of tyrosine-phosphorylated GAP for up to 8 hours following PDGF stimulation (data not shown).

GAP has previously been reported to be localized in the cell cytosol (Trahey and McCormick 1987). Our findings that GAP was rapidly tyrosine-phosphorylated in response to PDGF led us to perform subcellular fractionation studies to determine the site of GAP tyrosine phosphorylation within the cell. We found that in quiescent fibroblasts, GAP was predominantly localized in the soluble (cystolic) fraction. However, after stimulation of the cells with PDGF, we could observe a reproducible increase in membrane-associated GAP concomitant with a decrease in the cytosolic component. Furthermore, after anti-phosphotyrosine immunoprecipitation of each subcellular fraction, we observed tyrosine-phosphorylated GAP only in PDGF-stimulated cells that was most abundant in the membrane-enriched fraction. Thus, PDGFR activation induces a rapid tyrosine-phosphorylation of GAP that is localized in cell membranes (Molloy et al. 1989).

The rapid and sustained time course of GAP tyrosine phosphorylation is very similar to that recently reported for the PDGF-stimulated tyrosine phosphorylation of phospholipase C-γ (Meisenhelder et al. 1989). Furthermore, as with phospholipase C-γ, GAP has been shown to associate specifically with activated PDGFRs (Kazlauskas et al. 1990; C.J. Molloy, unpubl.). Taken together, these findings indicate that GAP is an early, direct substrate of the PDGFR tyrosine kinase.

Functional Significance of PDGF-induced Tyrosine Phosphorylation of GAP

Tyrosine phosphorylation is known to modulate the activity of a number of enzymes, including the *src* product (Hunter and Cooper 1985; Piwnica-Worms et al. 1987). It is also well established that a membrane localization for the *ras* p21 molecule is required for its biological activity (Willingham et al. 1980). Thus, the observation that tyrosine-phosphorylated GAP was predominantly associated with the cell membrane further suggests that tyrosine phosphorylation may alter the functional interaction of GAP and *ras* p21. In one proposed model, GAP serves as an attenuator of *ras* p21 function (McCormick 1989). If so, tyrosine phosphorylation of GAP may transiently remove its inhibition, allowing the *ras* p21-GTP complex to effect mitogenic signaling through some unknown downstream components. Another model suggests that GAP may act as a downstream effector and as attenuator of *ras* p21 function (Cales et al. 1988; McCormick 1989). Thus, tyrosine phosphorylation of GAP may modulate its effector role, perhaps by coupling the *ras* p21-GAP complex to other molecules. By whatever mechanism tyrosine phosphorylation may perturb *ras* p21-GAP function, these studies provide biochemical evidence linking these important growth regulatory molecules to the mitogenic signaling cascade that is activated by PDGF. Furthermore, these findings provide potentially critical targets for therapeutic intervention in human malignancies involving both autocrine-activated tyrosine kinases and mutated *ras* proteins.

REFERENCES

Betsholtz, C., A. Johnsson, C.-H. Heldin, and B. Westermark. 1986. Efficient reversion of simian sarcoma virus-transformation and inhibition of growth factor induced mitogenesis by suramin. *Proc. Natl. Acad. Sci.* **83:** 6440.

Cales, C., J.F. Hancock, C.J. Marshall, and A. Hall. 1988. The cytoplasmic protein GAP is implicated as the target for regulation by the ras gene product. *Nature* **332:** 548.

Doolittle, R.F., M.W. Hunkapiller, L.E. Hood, S.G. Devare, K.C. Robbins, S.A. Aaronson, and H.N. Antoniades. 1983. Simian sarcoma virus *onc* gene, v-*sis*, is derived from the gene (or genes) encoding a platelet-derived growth factor. *Science* **221:** 275.

Downward, J., Y. Yarden, E. Mayes, G. Scrace, N. Totty, P. Stockwell, A. Ullrich, J. Schlessinger, and M.D. Waterfield. 1984. Close similarity of epidermal growth factor receptor and v-*erb*-B oncogene protein sequences. *Nature* **307:** 521.

Farquhar, M.G. 1985. Progress in unraveling pathways of golgi traffic. *Annu. Rev. Cell Biol.* **1:** 447.

Fleming, T.P., T. Matsui, C.J. Molloy, K.C. Robbins, and S.A. Aaronson. 1989. Autocrine mechanism for v-*sis* transformation requires cell surface localization of internally activated growth factor receptors. *Proc. Natl. Acad. Sci.* **86:** 8063.

Gazit, A., H. Igarashi, I.-M. Chiu, A. Srinivasan, A. Yaniv, S. Tronick, K.C. Robbins, and S.A. Aaronson. 1984. Expression of the normal human *sis*/PDGF-2 coding sequence induces cellular transformation. *Cell* **39:** 89.

Gerwin, B.I., J.F. Lechner, R.R. Reddel, A.B. Roberts, K.C. Robbins, E.W. Gabrielson, and C.C. Harris. 1987. Comparison of production of transforming growth factor-β and platelet-derived growth factor by normal human mesothelial cells and mesothelial cell lines. *Cancer Res.* **47:** 6180.

Hannink, M. and D.J. Donoghue. 1988. Autocrine stimulation by the v-*sis* gene product requires a ligand-receptor interaction at the cell surface. *J. Cell Biol.* **107:** 287.

Heldin, C.-H. and B. Westermark. 1989. Platelet-derived growth factor-3 isoforms and two receptor types. *Trends Genet.* **5:** 108.

Huang, S.I., S.S. Huang, and T.F. Deuel. 1984. Transforming protein of simian sarcoma virus stimulates autocrine growth of SSV-transformed cells through PDGF cell-surface receptors. *Cell* **39:** 79.

Huang, S.S. and J.S. Huang. 1988. Rapid turnover of the platelet-derived growth factor receptor in *sis*-transformed cells and reversal by suramin. *J. Biol. Chem.* **263:** 12608.

Hunter, T. and J. Cooper. 1985. Protein-tyrosine kinases. *Annu. Rev. Biochem.* **54:** 897.

Johnsson, A., C. Betsholtz, C.-H. Heldin, and B. Westermark. 1985. Antibodies against platelet-derived growth factor inhibit acute transformation by simian sarcoma virus. *Nature* **317:** 438.

Kaplan, D.R., M. Whitman, B. Schaffhausen, D.C. Pallas, M. White, L. Cantley, and T.M. Roberts. 1987. Common elements in growth factor stimulation and oncogenic transformation: 85kd phosphoprotein and phosphatidylinositol kinase activity. *Cell* **50:** 1021.

Kazlauskas, A., C. Ellis, T. Pawson, and J.A. Cooper. 1990. Binding of GAP to activated PDGF receptor. *Science* **247:** 1578.

Keating, M.T. and L.T. Williams. 1988. Autocrine stimulation of intracellular PDGF receptors in v-*sis*-transformed cells. *Science* **239:** 914.

LaRocca, R.V., C.A. Stein, and C.E. Meyers. 1990. Suramin: Prototype of a new generation of antitumor compounds. *Cancer Cells* **2:** 106.

Leal, F., L.T. Williams, K.C. Robbins, and S.A. Aaronson. 1985. Evidence that the v-*sis* gene product transforms by interaction with the receptor for platelet-derived growth factor. *Science* **230:** 327.

Matsui, T., M. Heidaran, T. Miki, N. Popescu, W. La Rochelle, M. Kraus, J.H. Pierce, and S.A. Aaronson. 1989. Isolation of a novel receptor cDNA establishes the existence of two PDGF receptor genes. *Science* **243:** 800.

McCormick, F. 1989. *ras* GTPase activating protein: Signal transmitter and signal terminator. *Cell* **56:** 5.

Meisenhelder, J., P.-G. Suh, S.G. Rhee, and T. Hunter. 1989. Phospholipase C-γ is a substrate for the PDGF and EGF receptor protein tyrosine kinases *in vivo* and *in vitro*. *Cell* **57:** 1109.

Molloy, C.J., D. Bottaro, T.P. Fleming, M.S. Marshall, J.B. Gibbs, and S.A. Aaronson. 1989. PDGF induction of tyrosine phosphorylation of GTPase activating protein. *Nature* **342:** 711.

Morrison, D.K., D.R. Kaplan, J.A. Escobedo, U.R. Rapp, T.M. Roberts, and L.T. Williams. 1989. Direct activation of the serine/threonine kinase activity of Raf-1 through tyrosine phosphorylation by the PDGF-β receptor. *Cell* **58:** 649.

Mulcahy, L.S., M.R. Smith, and D.W. Stacey. 1985. Requirement for *ras* proto-oncogene function during serum-stimulated growth of NIH3T3 cells. *Nature* **313:** 241.

Piwnica-Worms, H., K.B. Saunders, T.M. Roberts, A.E. Smith, and S.H. Cheng. 1987. Tyrosine phosphorylation regulates the biochemical and biological properties of pp60$^{c\text{-}src}$. *Cell* **49:** 75.

Robbins, K.C., F. Leal, J.H. Pierce, and S.A. Aaronson. 1985. The v-*sis*/PDGF-2 transforming gene product localizes to cell membranes but is not a secretory protein. *EMBO J.* **4:** 1783.

Sherr, C.J., C.W. Rettenmier, R. Sacca, M.F. Roussel, A.T. Look, and E.R. Stanley. 1985. The c-*fms* proto-oncogene product is related to the receptor for the mononuclear phagocyte growth factor, CSF-1. *Cell* **41:** 665.

Sporn, M.B. and A.B. Roberts. 1985. Autocrine growth factors and cancer. *Nature* **313:** 745.

Trahey, M. and F. McCormick. 1987. A cytoplasmic protein stimulates normal N-*ras* p21 GTPase, but does not affect oncogenic mutants. *Science* **238:** 542.

Trahey, M., G. Wong, R. Halenbeck, B. Rubinfeld, G.A. Martin, M. Ladner, C.M. Long, W.J. Crosier, K. Watt, K. Koth, and F. McCormick. 1988. Molecular cloning of two types of GAP complementary DNA from human placenta. *Science* **242:** 1697.

Ullrich, A. and J. Schlessinger. 1990. Signal transduction by receptors with tyrosine kinase activity. *Cell* **61:** 203.

Versnel, M.A., A. Hagemeijer, M.J. Bouts, T.H. van der Kwast, and H.C. Hoogsteden. 1988. Expression of c-*sis* (PDGF-B chain) and PDGF-A chain genes in ten human malignant mesothelioma cell lines derived from primary and metastatic tumors. *Oncogene* **2:** 601.

Vogel, U.S., R.A.F. Dixon, M.D. Schaber, R.E. Diehl, M.S. Marshall, E.M. Scolnick, I.S. Sigal, and J.B. Gibbs. 1988. Cloning of bovine GAP and its interaction with oncogenic *ras* p21. *Nature* **335:** 90.

Wahl, M., N.E. Olashaw, S. Nishibe, S.G. Rhee, W.J. Pledger, and G. Carpenter. 1989. Platelet-derived growth factor induces rapid and sustained tyrosine phosphorylation of phospholipase C-γ in quiescent BALB/3T3 cells. *Mol. Cell Biol.* **9:** 2934.

Waterfield, M.D., G.T. Scrace, N. Whittle, P. Stroobant, A. Johnsson, A. Wasteson, B. Westermark, C.H. Heldin, J.S. Huang, and T.F. Deuel. 1983. Platelet-derived growth factor is structurally related to the putative transforming protein p28^{sis} of simian sarcoma virus. *Nature* **304:** 35.

Willingham, M.C., I. Pastan, T.Y. Shih, and E.M. Scolnick. 1980. Localization of the src gene product of the Harvey strain of MSV to plasma membrane of transformed cells by electron microscopic immunocytochemistry. *Cell* **19:** 1005.

Production of Cytokines by Particle-exposed Lung Macrophages

A.R. Brody

Laboratory of Pulmonary Pathobiology
National Institute of Environmental Health Sciences
Research Triangle Park, North Carolina 27709

INTRODUCTION

Lung disease caused by inhaling inorganic particles (i.e., pneumoconiosis) occurs commonly around the world (Selikoff and Lee 1978). Usually, the disease is manifested as a restrictive process wherein scar tissue deposition in the pulmonary interstitium leads to a stiff, noncompliant lung (Spencer 1977). The basic biological mechanisms through which inhalation of inorganic particles, such as silica and asbestos, cause interstitial pulmonary fibrosis (IPF) remain largely undefined (Brody et al. 1985). Although lung scarring can be induced by a variety of agents, the diseases caused by fibers have attracted a great deal of attention. This is because asbestos fibers have been shown to cause not only pneumoconiosis, but also lung cancer and mesothelioma (Craighead and Mossman 1982). In addition, asbestos fibers still are used for some commercial purposes and are found in buildings and schools in the millions of tons (Altree-Williams and Preston 1985). Thus, the likelihood of continued exposure to asbestos is high, and new technologies for producing man-made mineral fibers could add additional health risks (Lippman 1990).

To deal effectively with the diseases caused by naturally occurring and man-made mineral fibers, it is essential that we establish the basic biological, biochemical, and molecular mechanisms through which fibers cause cells to die, proliferate, migrate, or transform to a neoplastic phenotype. In this paper, we consider the biological activity of a group of polypeptide

Cellular and Molecular Aspects of Fiber Carcinogenesis
Copyright 1991 Cold Spring Harbor Laboratory Press 0-87969-361-4/91 $1.00 + 00

hormone-like cytokines collectively termed "growth factors" (Morstyn and Burgess 1988), particularly those factors synthesized and secreted by lung macrophages exposed to fibers.

Lung Macrophages

Since this book is not concerned primarily with lung macrophages, it should be useful to provide a brief background on this cell type. Pulmonary macrophages (PM) are large (15–30 μm) pleomorphic cells that possess phagocytic and lytic properties, and provide an effective defense against inhaled inorganic particles and microorganisms (Brody and Davis 1982). Pulmonary macrophages originate from bone-marrow-derived, blood-borne monocytes that differentiate in the lung (Van Furth and Cohn 1968). Macrophages, which are seen in the air spaces, may originate directly from the monocytes or from a local cell population within the interstitium of the lung (Brain et al. 1977). These interstitial macrophages may divide, dependent on such stimuli as increased phagocytic load (Bowden and Adamson 1972). Interstitial macrophages move through alveolar basement membranes and between alveolar lining cells during migration to the air spaces in both normal and pathologic tissues (Bowden and Adamson 1972; Davis et al. 1978). In the alveolar spaces, macrophages reside in a unique microenvironment, i.e., adherent to the alveolar surface, in humidified air, and bathed in the lipoproteins, enzymes, and serum constituents of the alveolar lining layer. The alveolar macrophage is a highly aerobic cell that is dependent on high-oxygen tensions and cannot phagocytize effectively in a hypoxic liquid environment where polymorphonuclear leukocytes and peritoneal macrophages carry on quite well (Green et al. 1977).

After a macrophage has entered an alveolar space, the pathways out of the lung are limited. The majority of PMs are carried from the lung by the mucociliary escalator to be swallowed or expectorated (Brody and Davis 1982). There is little direct experimental evidence to support the notion that macrophages reenter the interstitium from alveolar spaces in reverse of the interepithelial migration route (Harmson et al. 1985).

Thus, particle-macrophage interactions are likely to occur in both the air spaces and interstitium of the lung.

Macrophages ingest a variety of particles, as the primary phagocytes of the lung (Fig. 1). In this regard, many investigators have proposed that the lung macrophage is a major protagonist in mediating particle-induced lung disease (Brain 1980). Indeed, there are good reasons to implicate the macrophage. Historically, pathologists have recognized that macrophages form the nidus of a variety of pulmonary lesions, from tuberculous granulomas to talc- or silica-induced scars (Spencer 1977). Early studies in vitro showed that toxic particles, such as silica and asbestos, cause cell death (Chamberlain and Brown 1978). Concurrent studies in the 1960s and 1970s focused on the biology and biochemistry of an impressive array of macrophage-derived proteolytic enzymes that were

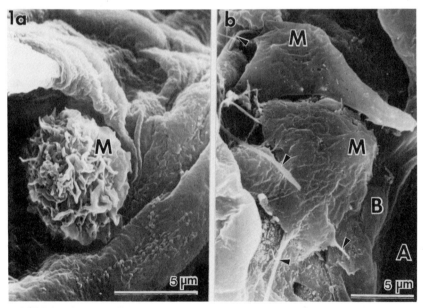

FIGURE 1 (a) Scanning electron micrography of a normal, ruffled macrophage (M) on the alveolar surface in the lung of an unexposed rat. Normally, macrophages are evenly distributed at about one or fewer per alveolar space. (b) Macrophages (M) accumulate at alveolar duct (AD) bifurcations (B) where numerous fibers (arrowheads) are phagocytized 48 hr after a 5-hr exposure to chrysotile asbestos.

thought to mediate fibrotic and/or emphysematous lung diseases (Allison 1977). Thus, it was logical to support the view that when inhaled toxic particles were phagocytized at the alveolar level, macrophage death ensued, and enzymes that were released caused the consequent pneumoconiosis. However, convincing evidence to support this concept has never been put forth. The alveolar surface is richly endowed with antiproteases, such as α_1-antiprotease and α_2-macroglobulin (α_2M) (Muller and vonWichert 1984). Thus, if the macrophage is indeed the cause of fibrotic lung disease, more subtle mediators will have to be sought. This brings us to the more modern view of how macrophages might control fibrogenesis after exposure to particles. Probably, to best understand how complex this theory must be, one should consult the review by Nathan (1987), which lists the "secretory products of macrophages." The list is astounding with more than 80 products within. Perhaps three groups of macrophage-derived secretions are most relevant to this discussion. The first-reactive oxygen species and the second-arachidonic acid metabolites are beyond the purview of this paper. Much has been written about these powerful mediators (Kouzan et al. 1985), and there is no question that they are central to many cellular events in the lung such as epithelial necrosis and control of fibroblast proliferation (Elias et al. 1985). A third group of macrophage products to consider are collectively termed "cytokines" (Tovey 1988). Little is known about their putative role in the pathogenesis of lung disease, and less is known about which of the factors might be produced by fiber-exposed macrophages. A review of this relatively new field constitutes the remainder of this discussion.

Particle-exposed Lung Macrophages

Kelley (1990), in his excellent review of lung cytokines, provides a chapter on macrophage-derived cytokines. The major cytokines included in his list are platelet-derived growth factor (PDGF), interleukin-1 (IL-1) and interleukin-6 (IL-6), tumor necrosis factor-α (TNF-α), transforming growth factor-β (TGF-β), fibroblast growth factor, and insulin-like growth factor-1 (IGF-1). As early as 1922 (Carrel 1922) and more recently in the 1970s (Leibovich and Ross 1975, 1976), investigators recognized that macrophages are capable of producing materials that stimulate mesenchymal cells to migrate and proliferate. These studies form the cornerstone of the current hypothesis, which states that mesenchymal growth factors from macrophages can mediate interstitial fibrogenesis. Now that the biological potentials of the various growth factors are more clear, it is not surprising that the macrophage secretions studied in "conditioned medium" are good stimulators of cell growth. For example, PDGF has been shown to be a most potent enhancer of mesenchymal cell proliferation (Ross et al. 1986), and Shimokado et al. (1985) demonstrated that lung macrophages secrete PDGF and that this factor accounts for more than 60% of the macrophage-derived mitogenic activity. Similarly, IGF-1 has been elegantly studied by Rom et al. (1988). IGF-1 is secreted by lung macrophages, was originally identified as alveolar macrophage-derived growth factor (Bitterman et al. 1982), and serves as an excellent "progression factor" for cell proliferation. If one applies the concepts of "competence" and "progression" in the control of mesenchymal cell proliferation (Gillespie et al. 1985), it is clear how macrophage-conditioned medium provides both in the form of PDGF and IGF-1, respectively.

What is the evidence that fiber-exposed macrophages secrete the cytokines discussed above and that these products play any role in the pathogenesis of pulmonary fibrosis? Evidence for secretion is very good (Kelley 1990); evidence for a causal role remains circumstantial. First, let us consider what is known about production.

A series of studies from the National Institute of Health has shown that macrophages from the lungs of patients with IPF secrete increased amounts of PDGF (Bitterman et al. 1983, 1986). Populations of individuals exposed to fibrogenic dusts, such as silica and asbestos, also exhibited increased levels of macrophage-derived PDGF (Rom et al. 1987). There are few studies on the production of cytokines by cells from the lungs of experimental animals exposed to particles. Driscoll et al. (1990) used intratracheal instillation of silica and titanium dioxide (TiO_2) to induce macrophages to produce IL-1 and TNF. Schmidt et al. (1984) showed that silica-stimulated monocytes produce IL-1, and Hartmann et al. (1984) demonstrated production of the same cytokine after asbestos inhalation. Lemaire et al. (1986) were the first to claim that asbestos induced the production of "factors" that were able to control fibroblast proliferation. Unfortunately, the factors were not defined in their model and could have been any of a number of the macrophage-derived products described above.

Our studies on asbestos-exposed animals have used brief exposures to aerosols of chrysotile asbestos fibers (Brody and Hill 1982). The object of our investigations is to establish the basic biological, biochemical, and molecular mechanisms through which inhaled fibers cause a progressive fibrogenic lung disease. Earlier studies showed that the fibers initially were deposited at the bifurcations of alveolar ducts (Brody and Roe 1983). These fibers activated alveolar complement through the alternative pathway producing a cleavage product of the fifth component of complement, C5a (Warheit et al. 1985), and this potent chemotactic factor attracted macrophages to the alveolar duct bifurcations where the fibers were phagocytized both on the alveolar surfaces and in the interstitium (Brody and Hill 1982; Warheit et al. 1986) (Fig. 1). Macrophage accumulation ensued over 72 hours, following a single, brief exposure (Warheit et al. 1986). Most interesting in this regard was the finding that, during the macrophage response, a variety of cell types in and around the bronchiolar-alveolar duct junctions exhibited dramatic increases in incorporation of tritiated thymidine ([^{3}H]TdR]) (Fig. 2) (Brody and Overby 1989). Lung cells normally have a low turnover rate, which is usually less than 1% (Evans and Bils 1969). Asbestos induced 10- to 20-fold increases in [^{3}H]TdR incorporation by bronchiolar and alveolar epithelial cells, interstitial fibroblasts, and myofibroblasts, as well as endothelial and smooth muscle cells of small pulmonary vessels (McGavran et al. 1990) (Fig. 2). All of these increases were found only in cells of the bronchiolar-alveolar duct (BAD) junctions (Brody and Overby 1989); random sections through the lung revealed no increases in the general parenchyma (Brody and Overby 1989), and inhalation of nonfibrogenic iron spheres also caused no [^{3}H]TdR incorporation (Brody and Overby 1989). Studies using ultrastructural morphometry showed that the increased [^{3}H]TdR

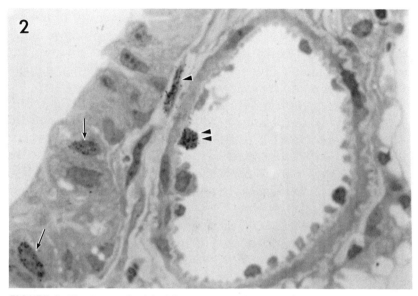

FIGURE 2 Plastic-embedded lung tissue from the lung of a mouse 48 hr after a 3-hr exposure to chrysotile asbestos. Bronchiolar epithelial cells (arrows), interstitial fibroblasts (arrowhead), and a vascular endothelial cell (double arrowheads) have incorporated [³H]TdR into DNA as a result of asbestos exposure. (For further details, see Brody and Overby 1989; McGavran et al. 1990.)

uptake resulted in highly significant increases in cell volume and number at the BAD junctions (Chang et al. 1988), and smooth muscle cells of the small vessels were thicker and doubled in number at 1-month postexposure (McGavran et al. 1990). Morphometry also demonstrated that the bifurcations were increased in volume because of excess connective tissue matrix (Chang et al. 1988). Considered together, these findings have led us to form the central hypothesis that a variety of diffusible "growth factors" are elicited consequent to asbestos exposure. Which factors are significant and which cells produce them in the developing lesions are obvious objects of ongoing investigations. Inasmuch as macrophages comprise a significant component of the asbestos-induced lesions, and since these cells are capable of producing a broad spectrum of such factors (as discussed above), we are studying growth factor production by lung macrophages in vitro and in vivo.

It is clear that the list of macrophage-derived growth factors is very long (Nathan 1987), and it is not wise to try to investigate all the possibilities. Why, then, have we opted to study PDGF and TGF-β? As described above and in an excellent review (Ross et al. 1986), PDGF is the most potent mitogen that is known for mesenchymal cells. Similarly, TGF-β has been shown to be a powerful inducer of extracellular matrix production by fibroblasts (Raghow et al. 1987; Sporn et al. 1987). Inasmuch as cell proliferation and matrix production are prominent features of asbestos-induced lung disease, PDGF and TGF-β are reasonable candidates for close scrutiny.

First, it was necessary that we establish whether or not rat lung macrophages synthesize and secrete PDGF. These cells do indeed produce PDGF, as determined by a quantitative enzyme immunoassay developed in our laboratory (Kumar et al. 1988a,b). It was interesting to learn that a goat anti-human PDGF antibody (Collaborative Research, Lexington, Massachusetts) cross-reacted with rat PDGF and allowed us to identify the rat macrophage-derived (MD) PDGF that had been fractionated from macrophage-conditioned culture medium (MCM) by high-pressure liquid chromatography (HPLC) (Fig. 3). As discussed above, the MCM can act as a growth-promoting medium for mesenchymal cells, since macrophages secrete a variety of components that support cell growth. When macrophages were exposed to a variety of particles, the growth-promoting capacity of the MCM increased significantly (Bauman et al. 1990). Interestingly enough, zymosan particles initially caused a burst of growth factor secretion by macrophages during the first 4 hours of culture (Bauman et al. 1990). This effect diminished with time and had returned to control levels after 24 hours of culture. In contrast, iron spheres and asbestos fibers were slower in inducing growth factor activity by macrophages, but the effect was still significantly above control levels after the 48-hour culture period (Bauman et al. 1990). We postulated that the maintenance of growth factor release was due to the nondegradable nature of the particles that continued to stimulate the macrophages through mechanisms not yet established (Gallagher et al. 1987; Scheule and Holian 1990). We hoped to identify the growth factor, and since the MCM is so complex, it was neces-

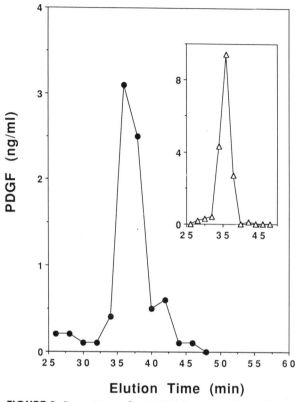

FIGURE 3 Secretion of a PDGF homolog by asbestos-stimulated rat alveolar macrophages. Macrophages obtained by saline lavage were allowed to adhere to a plastic tissue culture surface for 45 min in serum-free Dulbecco's modified Eagle's medium (37°C/5% CO_2 humidified air) and then were exposed to chrysotile asbestos (15 $\mu g/cm^2$) for 24 hr. The macrophage-conditioned medium was concentrated 100x using a 5-kD cutoff filter, acidified to 1 M acetic acid, and loaded onto a Superose 12 FPLC (Pharmacia) column that was equilibrated to 1 M acetic acid. Column fractions were neutralized with Tris, and PDGF was measured by an enzyme immunoassay that relies on a monospecific antibody raised against human PDGF. The same immunoassay was used to detect human PDGF that was used as a standard reference (*inset*). Chromatograms courtesy of Dr. J.C. Bonner, Laboratory of Pulmonary Pathology, National Institute of Environmental Health Sciences, Research Triangle Park, North Carolina. For further details, see Bonner et al. (1989, 1990).

sary to separate the medium by HPLC and to characterize those fractions by biological and biochemical assays. These studies resulted in two major findings: (1) the discovery of a MD binding protein for PDGF (Bonner et al. 1989) and (2) the chemotactic nature of MD-PDGF for rat lung fibroblasts (RLFs) (Osornio-Vargas et al. 1990).

Binding Proteins for PDGF

In 1984, Huang et al. (1984) showed that some of the PDGF in serum was bound to α_2M, a high-molecular-weight (~700 kD) antiprotease (Sottrup-Jensen 1989). They suggested that the binding protein would aid in the clearance of PDGF from serum and fluids. Now, we have shown that lung macrophages exposed to iron spheres and asbestos fibers secrete increased levels of PDGF, about 50% of which is bound to macrophage-derived α_2M (Bonner et al. 1989). This antiprotease can be found in a native or "slow" form, and after interaction with a wide variety of proteases, the α_2M becomes receptor-recognized and is termed the "fast" form because of its relatively faster migration on polyacrylamide gels (Sottrup-Jensen 1989). MD-PDGF binds to both the slow and fast forms (Bonner et al. 1989). It was fascinating to learn that when the PDGF is bound to receptor-recognized α_2M, it stimulates the proliferation of lung fibroblasts by more than 100% over PDGF alone (Bonner et al. 1990). The slow form of α_2M blocks PDGF proliferation at higher concentrations, and at lower concentrations fibroblast-derived proteases convert the α_2M to a fast form that enhances fibroblast growth (Bonner et al. 1990). Since this fibroblast growth can be blocked by anti-PDGF antibodies, we suggest that the α_2M, which is bound to its receptor on the fibroblast membrane, allows more PDGF to reach its own receptor on the cell surface. The result is enhanced fibroblast proliferation. This could be a potentially significant mechanism that controls local concentrations of PDGF, and studies are ongoing to establish whether or not this complex would be effective in vivo.

Fibroblast Chemotaxis to PDGF

As discussed above, accumulation of lung fibroblasts and their products is a hallmark of fibrotic lung disease. The mechan-

isms through which the fibroblasts increase in the lung interstitium probably are twofold: proliferation, as described above,
and chemotaxis. Chemotaxis, i.e., the directed migration of
cells to a chemical signal, is a characteristic of numerous cell
types (Zigmond and Hirsch 1973). From the lung, epithelial
cells (Shoji et al. 1990), fibroblasts (Osornio-Vargas et al.
1990), macrophages (Warheit et al. 1985), and other inflammatory cells (Donaldson et al. 1990) have been shown to
respond to a variety of chemotactic factors. Among the most
potent chemotactic factors are several of the cytokines
(Grotendorst and Martin 1986). We have reasoned that if macrophages produce chemotactic factors for lung fibroblasts, an
additional mechanism controlling fibroblast accumulation
could be operating after macrophage activation. Since PDGF
has been shown to be chemotactic for mesenchymal cells,
such as smooth muscle cells (Martinet et al. 1987) and fibroblast cell lines (Grotendorst 1984), we investigated whether the
rat macrophage-derived PDGF was chemotactic for RLFs. We
found (Osornio-Vargas et al. 1990) that purified human PDGF
and the MD-PDGF were chemotactic for early-passage RLFs
but not for lung macrophages. RLFs exhibited a typical bell-
shaped, dose-related curve and responded optimally between 2
and 4 ng/ml PDGF. Alveolar macrophage-conditioned medium
(AMCM), fractionated by gel filtration in 1 M acetic acid, induced a clear chemotactic response in the same fractions
(20–22 ml), where PDGF was identified by enzyme immunoassay. In contrast, AMCM fractionated by gel filtration in
phosphate-buffered saline (PBS) did not induce any chemotactic activity unless the fractions were treated further with 1 M
acetic acid. In this case, chemotactic activity was observed in
those fractions with molecular masses of 150 kD and >200
kD. All chemotactic activity observed with fractionated AMCM
was blocked >90% by an anti-PDGF antibody. These observations demonstrate that MD-PDGF is chemotactic for RLFs if it
first is released from its binding protein, α-macroglobulin (αM),
which is secreted into the medium along with PDGF (Bonner et
al. 1989). Thus, additional experiments were carried out to
test whether or not bovine α_2M, a plasma homolog of the
macrophage-derived αM, modulated the chemotactic activity of
human PDGF. Bovine α_2M caused a concentration-dependent

inhibition of PDGF-induced chemotaxis. This correlates with our finding of no chemotactic activity in the high-molecular-weight regions of fractionated conditioned medium, unless the macrophage-derived binding protein was removed by acidification. These findings demonstrated the potent chemotactic activity of PDGF for primary RLFs and emphasize the importance of binding proteins in modulating biological activity. Of course, we do not yet know whether or not the growth factor and its binding protein are active in vivo. Another important issue is our finding that the PDGF-related chemotactic activity could not be detected unless the macrophages first were stimulated by phagocytosis of iron spheres (Osornio-Vargas et al. 1990). We have some evidence that PDGF production by macrophages is up-regulated by phagocytosis of iron and asbestos fibers after the cells were exposed in vitro or in vivo (R.M. Schapira et al., in prep.). It will be essential to establish whether or not the chemotactic activity of PDGF is expressed during disease progression, since this could be a significant mechanism for increasing the population of interstitial lung fibroblasts.

Production of TGF-β

The emphasis in our laboratory has been on control of fibroblast proliferation in a "positive" sense, i.e., induction of proliferation. However, it is very clear that such proliferative events of fibroblasts must have negative or inhibitory controls (Reiser and Last 1986) and that the fibroblasts produce increased amounts of extracellular matrix components both in vitro and in vivo (Goldstein and Fine 1986). An extremely potent inhibitor of mesenchymal cell proliferation and stimulator of matrix production is TGF-β (Roberts and Sporn 1988).

TGF-β is a 25-kD protein secreted by both normal and transformed cells and has been characterized by its ability to reversibly induce anchorage-independent growth of non-transformed cells (Roberts and Sporn 1988). TGF-β consists of at least two distinct but structurally related forms: TGF-β1 and TGF-β2. These are multifunctional agents capable of either stimulating or inhibiting proliferation of a multitude of cell types, as well as having profound effects on the synthesis and secretion of many components of the extracellular matrix (ECM) and on cell differentiation (Ignotz and Massague 1986; Roberts and Sporn 1988). Modulation of cell growth and stimulation of ECM production by TGF-β in several types of normal and transformed fibroblastic cell lines have been reported previously (Roberts and Sporn 1988). These important biological properties have been shown in an embryonic lung fibroblast cell line (Hill et al. 1986) and in fibroblasts obtained from normal adult human lungs (Fine and Goldstein 1987). In addition, TGF-β has been demonstrated by immunochemistry techniques in the lungs of animals treated with the fibrogenic agent bleomycin (Khalil et al. 1989).

Numerous cell types tested have been shown to possess specific high-affinity receptors for TGF-β (Roberts and Sporn 1988) with a range of binding-affinity dissociation constants (K_d) of 1–100 pM and variable numbers of receptors (1,000–80,000 per cell). Three distinct types of TGF-β glycoprotein receptor molecules with different molecular weight ranges have been identified using affinity-labeling techniques (Roberts and Sporn 1988). These have been designated as type I $(M_r = 50,000–80,000)$, type II $(M_r = 85,000–140,000)$, and type III $(M_r = 250,000–330,000)$. The pattern of TGF-β binding to different cells is variable, since some cells lack the type III receptor protein but remain responsive to TGF-β.

Using a procedure for obtaining normal primary RLFs and maintaining these cells in culture, we established the binding kinetics and receptor subunit structures for both ^{125}I-labeled TGF-β1 and ^{125}I-labeled TGF-β2 under identical conditions (Kalter and Brody 1991). In these experiments, we demonstrated that the RLF TGF-β receptor exhibits different affinities for TGF-β1 and TGF-β2 in both homologous and heterologous ligand-receptor studies of the two TGF-βs. The data demonstrate that the biological potency of TGF-β1 is greater than that of TGF-β2 in growth inhibition studies (Kalter and Brody 1991). This was the first demonstration of biologically responsive TGF-β receptors with different affinities for TGF-β1 and TGF-β2 on normal, nonimmortal fibroblastic cells derived from adult rat lung. In addition, we have presented the first evidence for the secretion of a TGF-β-like molecule by rat alveolar macrophages (AM) in vitro (Kalter et al. 1989). This macrophage-derived TGF-β binds to both TGF-β1 and TGF-β2 receptors on the RLFs. Furthermore, secretion of this TGF-β activity can be enhanced by exposure of AM to carbonyl iron spheres in vitro.

There is a single class of high-affinity receptors (~10,000 sites/cell) for TGF-β1 (K_d = 23 pM) and TGF-β2 (K_d = 41 pM) on early passage RLFs (Kalter and Brody 1991). Incubation with unlabeled TGF-β1 and TGF-β2 resulted in concentration-dependent inhibition of binding of ^{125}I-labeled TGF-β1 (ED_{50} = 20 pM and 28 pM) and ^{125}I-labeled TGF-β2 (ED_{50} = 36 pM and 56 pM). Overnight incubation with 400 pM TGF-β induced down-regulation of TGF-β1 and TGF-β2 binding sites. TGF-β receptors affinity cross-linked with 100 pM ^{125}I-labeled TGF-β1 or ^{125}I-labeled TGF-β2 were subjected to SDS-polyacrylamide gel electrophoresis and exhibited labeled protein bands of 68 kD, 88 kD, and 286 kD. Densitometric analysis of the resulting autoradiograms showed that the labeled bands exhibited different affinities for the two forms of TGF-β (Kalter and Brody 1991). TGF-β1 was more potent than TGF-β2 in the inhibition of RLF growth, with 50% inhibition by 0.12 pM TGF-β1 and 4.4 pM TGF-β2. These data demonstrate the production of a fibrogenic cytokine (TGF-β) by rat lung macrophages and the presence of specific TGF-β receptors on nonimmortal putative target cells (lung fibroblasts). These observations support the concept that macrophage-derived growth factors could play a central role in pulmonary fibrogenesis.

SUMMARY AND CONCLUSIONS

It seems reasonable to speculate that lung macrophages provide the factors that mediate interstitial lung disease. All the necessary components have been demonstrated in vitro. However, none has been proven to play any role in the lungs in vivo in humans or animals. Recent studies showing clear effects of PDGF and TGF-β on wound healing (Greenhalgh et al. 1990) and amelioration of silicosis by anti-TNF antibodies support the postulate (Piguet et al. 1990). Thus, we are at the juncture where most (if not all) of the significant growth factors probably have been discovered and characterized (at least in part). Now, we must carry out the experiments, which will allow us to establish which factors are mediating the disease process and the biochemical and molecular mechanisms through which the factors operate.

It is clear that particle-exposed macrophages produce increased amounts of the factors discussed above. The mechanism(s) through which particles such as asbestos fibers and inorganic and organic spheres cause this stimulation are unknown. The biology, biochemistry, and molecular nature of the growth factor receptors have not been studied after the membranes have been perturbed by particles and fibers. Such investigations could be essential in furthering our understanding of particle-induced lung disease.

ACKNOWLEDGMENTS

The author is indebted to Drs. James C. Bonner, Valerie G. Kalter, and Alvaro Osornio-Vargas, who currently are carrying this work forward in the laboratory. I also thank Ms. Lynne Moore for preparation of Figures 1 and 2. The animal inhalation facility is operated under a contract to Northrop Services, Inc., whose continuous cooperation is greatly appreciated.

REFERENCES

Allison, A.C. 1977. Mechanisms of macrophage toxicity in relation to the pathogenesis of some lung diseases. In *Respiratory defense mechanisms* (ed. J.D. Brain et al.), vol. 2, p. 1075. Marcel Dekker, New York.

Altree-Williams, S. and J.S. Preston. 1985. Asbestos and other fiber levels in buildings. *Ann. Occup. Hyg.* **29:** 357.

Bauman, M.D., A.M. Jetten, J.C. Bonner, R.K. Kumar, R.A. Bennett, and A.R. Brody. 1990 Secretion of a platelet-derived growth factor homologue by rat alveolar macrophages exposed to particulates in vitro. *Eur. J. Cell Biol.* **51:** 327.

Bitterman, P.B., S. Adelberg, and R.G. Crystal. 1983. Mechanisms of pulmonary fibrosis. Spontaneous release of the alveolar macrophage-derived growth factor in the interstitial lung disorders. *J. Clin. Invest.* **72:** 1801.

Bitterman, P.B., S.I. Rennard, G.W. Hunninghake, and R.G. Crystal. 1982. Human alveolar macrophage growth factor for fibroblasts: Regulation and partial characterization. *J. Clin. Invest.* **70:** 806.

Bitterman P.B., S.I. Rennard, B.A. Keogh, M.D. Wewers, S. Adelberg, and R.G. Crystal. 1986. Familial idiopathic pulmonary fibrosis. Evidence of lung inflammation in unaffected family members. *N. Engl. J. Med.* **314:** 1343.

Bonner, J.C., M. Hoffman, and A.R. Brody. 1989. Alpha-macroglobulin secreted by alveolar macrophages serves as a binding protein for a macrophage-derived homologue of platelet-derived growth factor. *Am. J. Respir. Cell Mol. Biol.* **1:** 171.

Bonner, J.C., A. Badgett, A.R. Osornio-Vargas, M. Hoffman, and A.R. Brody. 1990. PDGF-stimulated fibroblast proliferation is enhanced synergistically by receptor recognized α_2-macroglobulin. *J. Cell Physiol.* **145:** 1.

Bowden, D.H., and I.Y.R. Adamson. 1972. The pulmonary interstitial cell as immediate precursor of the alveolar macrophage. *Am. J. Pathol.* **68:** 521.

Brain, J.D. 1980. Macrophage damage in relation to the pathogenesis of lung diseases. *Environ. Health Perspect.* **35:** 21.

Brain, J.D., J.J. Godleski, and S.P. Sorokin. 1977. Quantification, origin, and fate of pulmonary macrophages. In *Respiratory defense mechanisms* (ed. J.D. Brain et al.), p. 849. Marcel Dekker, New York.

Brody, A.R. and G.S. Davis. 1982. Alveolar macrophage toxicology. In *Mechanisms in respiratory toxicology* (ed. H. Witschi and P. Nettesheim), p. 3. CRC Press, Boca Raton, Florida.

Brody, A.R. and L.H. Hill. 1982. Interstitial accumulation of inhaled chrysotile asbestos fibers and consequent formation of microcalcifications. *Am. J. Pathol.* **109:** 107.

Brody, A.R. and L.H. Overby. 1989. Incorporation of tritiated thymidine by epithelial cells in bronchiolar-alveolar regions of asbestos exposed rats. *Am. J. Pathol.* **134:** 133.

Brody, A.R. and M.W. Roe. 1983. Deposition pattern of inorganic particles at the alveolar level in the lungs of rats and mice. *Am. Rev. Respir. Dis.* **128:** 724.

Brody, A.R., L.H. Hill, and D.B. Warheit. 1985. Induction of early alveolar injury by inhaled asbestos and silica. *Fed. Proc.* **44:** 2596.

Brody, A.R., L.H. Hill, B. Adkins, and R.W. O'Connor, Jr. 1981. Chrysotile asbestos inhalation in rats: Deposition pattern and reaction of alveolar epithelium and pulmonary macrophages. *Am. Rev. Respir. Dis.* **123:** 670.

Carrel, A. 1922. Growth-promoting function of leucocytes. *J. Exp. Med.* **35:** 385.

Chamberlain, M. and R.C. Brown. 1978. The cytotoxic effects of asbestos and other mineral dust in tissue culture cell lines. *Br. J. Exp. Pathol.* **59:** 183.

Chang, L.Y., L.H. Overby, A.R. Brody, and J.D. Crapo. 1988. Progressive lung cell reactions and extracellular matrix production after a brief exposure to asbestos. *Am. J. Pathol.* **131:** 156.

Craighead, J.E. and B.T. Mossman. 1982. The pathogenesis of asbestos-associated diseases. *N. Engl. J. Med.* **306:** 1446.

Davis, G.S., A.R. Brody and J.E. Craighead. 1978. Analysis of airspace and interstitial mononuclear cell populations in human diffuse interstitial lung disease. *Am. Rev. Respir. Dis.* **118:** 7.

Donaldson, K., G.M. Brown, D.M. Brown, J. Slight, M.D. Robertson, and J.M. Davis. 1990. Impaired chemotactic responses of bronchoalveolar leukocytes in experimental pneumoconiosis. *J. Pathol.* **160:** 63.

Driscoll, K.E., R.C. Linderschmidt, J.K. Maurer, J.M. Higgins, and G. Ridder. 1990. Pulmonary response to silica or titanium dioxide: Inflammatory cells, alveolar macrophage-derived cytokines, and histopathology. *Am. J. Resp. Cell Mol. Biol.* **2:** 381.

Elias, J.A., M.D. Rossman, R.B. Zurier, and R.P. Daniele. 1985. Human alveolar macrophage inhibition of lung fibroblast growth: A prostaglandin dependent process. *Am. Rev. Respir. Dis.* **131:** 94.

Evans, M.J. and R.F. Bils. 1969. Identification of cells labeled with tritiated thymidine in the pulmonary alveolar walls of the mouse. *Am. Rev. Respir. Dis.* **100:** 372.

Fine, A. and R.H. Goldstein. 1987. The effect of transforming growth factors on cell proliferation and collagen formation by lung fibroblasts. *J. Biol. Chem.* **262:** 3897.

Gallagher, J.E., G. George, and A.R. Brody. 1987. Sialic acid mediates the initial binding of positively charged inorganic particles to alveolar macrophage membranes. *Am. Rev. Respir. Dis.* **135:** 1345.

Gillespie, G.Y., J.E. Estes, and W.J. Pledger. 1985. Macrophage-derived growth factors for mesenchymal cells. In *Lymphokines* (ed. E. Pick), vol. 2, p. 213. Academic Press, Orlando, Florida.

Goldstein, R.H. and A. Fine. 1986. Fibrotic reactions in the lung: The activation of the lung fibroblast. *Exp. Lung Res.* **11:** 245.

Green, G.M., F.J. Jakab, R.B. Low, and G.S. Davis. 1977. Defense mechanisms of the respiratory membrane. *Am. Rev. Respir. Dis.* **115:** 479.

Greenhalgh, D.G., K.H. Sprugel, M.J. Murray, and R. Ross. 1990. PDGF and FGF stimulate wound healing in the genetically diabetic mouse. *Am. J. Pathol.* **136:** 1235.

Grotendorst, G.R. 1984. Alteration of the chemotactic response of NIH/3T3 cells to PDGF by growth factors, transformation and tumor promoters. *Cell* **36:** 279.

Grotendorst, G.R. and G.R. Martin. 1986. Cell movements in wound-healing and fibrosis. *Rheumatology* **10:** 385.

Harmson, A.G., B.A. Muggenberg, M.B. Snipes, and D.E. Bice. 1985. The role of macrophages in particle translocation from lung to lymph nodes. *Science* **230:** 1277.

Hartmann, D.P., M.M. Georgian, Y. Oghiso, and E. Kagan. 1984. Enhanced interleukin activity following asbestos inhalation. *Clin. Exp. Immunol.* **55:** 643.

Hill, D.J., S.F. Elstrow, I. Swenne, and R.D.G. Milner. 1986. Bifunctional action of transforming growth factor-β on DNA synthesis in early passage human fetal fibroblasts. *J. Cell Physiol.* **128:** 3222.

Huang, J.S., S.S. Huang, and T.S. Deuel. 1984. Specific covalent binding of platelet-derived growth factor to human plasma α_2-macroglobulin. *Proc. Natl. Acad. Sci.* **81:** 342.

Ignotz, R. and J. Massague. 1986. Transforming growth factor beta stimulates the expression of fibronectin and collagen and their incorporation into the extracellular matrix. *J. Biol. Chem.* **261:** 4337.

Kalter, V.G. and A.R. Brody. 1991. Receptors for TGFβ on rat lung fibroblasts have higher affinity for TGFβ1 than TGFβ2. *Am. J. Respir. Cell Mol. Biol.* (in press).

Kalter, V.G., J.C. Bonner, and A.R. Brody. 1989. Secretion of TGFβ by rat alveolar macrophages and characterization of TGFβ receptors on rat lung fibroblasts. *Cytokine* **1:** 76.

Kelley, J. 1990. Cytokines of the lung. *Am. Rev. Resp. Dis.* **141:** 765.

Khalil, N., O. Bereznay, M. Sporn, and A.H. Greenberg. 1989. Macrophage production of transforming growth factors and fibroblast collagen synthesis in chronic pulmonary inflammation. *J. Exp. Med.* **170:** 727.

Kouzan, S., A.R. Brody, P. Nettesheim, and T.E. Eling. 1985. Production of arachidonic acid metabolites by macrophages exposed in vitro to asbestos fibers, carbonyl iron, and calcium inophore. *Am. Rev. Respir. Dis.* **131:** 624.

Kumar, R.K., R.A. Bennett, and A.R. Brody. 1988a. A homologue of platelet-derived growth factor produced by alveolar macrophages. *FASEB J.* **2:** 2272.

––––––. 1988b. An enzyme immunoassay for platelet-derived growth factor: Application to the measurement of macrophage-derived PDGF. In *Monokines and other non-lymphocytic cytokines* (ed. C. Dinarello and M. Powanda), p. 393. A.R. Liss, New York.

Leibovich, S.J. and R. Ross. 1975. The role of the macrophage in wound repair. A study with hydrocortisone and antimacrophage serum. *Am. J. Pathol.* **78:** 71.

––––––. 1976. A macrophage-dependent factor that stimulates the proliferation of fibroblasts in vitro. *Am. J. Pathol.* **84:** 501.

Lemaire, I., H. Beaudoin, S. Masse, and C. Grondin. 1986. Alveolar macrophage stimulation of lung fibroblast growth in asbestos-induced pulmonary fibrosis. *Am. J. Pathol.* **122:** 205.

Lippman, M. 1990. Man-made mineral fibers: Human exposures and health risk assessment. *Toxicol. Ind. Health* **6:** 225.

Martinet, Y.M., W.N. Rom, G.R. Grotendorst, G.R. Martin, and R.G. Crystal. 1987. Exaggerated spontaneous release of platelet-derived growth factor by alveolar macrophages from patients with idiopathic pulmonary fibrosis. *N. Engl. J. Med.* **317:** 202.

McGavran, P.D., L.B. Moore, and A.R. Brody. 1990. Inhalation of chrysotile asbestos rapid cellular proliferation in small pulmonary vessels of mice and rats. *Am. J. Pathol.* **136:** 695.

Morstyn, G. and A.W. Burgess. 1988. Hemopoetic growth factors. A review. *Cancer Res.* **2:** 87.

Muller, B. and P. vonWichert. 1984. Identical serum proteins and specific bronchoalveolar lavage proteins in the adult human and rat. *Am. Rev. Respir. Dis.* **130:** 674.

Nathan, C.F. 1987. Secretory products of macrophages. *J. Clin. Invest.* **79:** 319.

Osornio-Vargas, A.R., J.C. Bonner, A. Badgett, and A.R. Brody. 1990. Rat alveolar macrophage-derived PDGF is chemotactic for rat lung fibroblasts. *Am. J. Resp. Cell Mol. Biol.* **3:** 595.

Piguet, P.F., M.A., Collart, G. Grav, A.P. Sappino, and P. Vassalli. 1990. Requirement of TNF for development of silica-induced pulmonary fibrosis. *Nature* **344:** 245.

Raghow, R., A.H. Kang, and D. Pidikiti. 1987. Phenotypic plasticity of extracellular matrix gene expression in cultured hamster lung fibroblasts. Regulation of type I procollagen and fibronectin synthesis. *J. Cell Biol.* **262:** 8409.

Reiser, K.M. and J.A. Last. 1986. Early cellular events in pulmonary fibrosis. *Exp. Lung Res.* **10:** 331.

Roberts, A.B. and M.B. Sporn. 1988. Transforming growth factor β. *Adv. Cancer Res.* **51:** 107.

Rom, W.N., P.B. Bitterman, S.I. Rennard, A. Cantin, and R.G. Crystal. 1987. Characterization of the lower respiratory tract inflammation of nonsmoking individuals with interstitial lung disease associated with chronic inhalation of inorganic dusts. *Am. Rev. Respir. Dis.* **136:** 1429.

Rom, W.N., P. Basset, G.A. Fells, T. Nukiwa, B.C. Trapnell, and R.G. Crystal. 1988. Alveolar macrophages release an insulin-like growth factor I-type molecule. *J. Clin. Invest.* **82:** 1685.

Ross, R., E.W. Raines, and D.G. Bowen-Pope. 1986. The biology of platelet-derived growth factor. *Cell* **46:** 155.

Scheule, R.K. and A. Holian. 1990. Modification of asbestos bioactivity for the alveolar macrophage by selective protein adsorption. *Am. J. Resp. Cell Mol. Biol.* **2:** 441.

Schmidt, J.A., C.N. Oliver, J.L. Lepe-Zuniga, I. Green, and I. Gery. 1984. Silica-stimulated monocytes release fibroblast proliferation factors identical to interleukin 1: A potential role for interleukin 1 in the pathogenesis of silicosis. *J. Clin. Invest.* **73:** 1462.

Selikoff, I.J. and D.H. Lee. 1978. *Asbestos and disease.* Academic Press, New York.

Shimokado, K., W.W. Raines, K.K. Madtes, T.B. Barrett, E.P. Benditt, and R. Ross. 1985. A significant part of macrophage-derived growth factor consists of at least two forms of PDGF. *Cell* **43:** 277.

Shoji, S., R.F. Ertl, J. Linder, S. Koizumi, W.C. Duckworth, and S.I. Rennard. 1990. Bronchial epithelial cells respond to insulin and insulin-like growth factor-I as a chemoattractant. *Am. J. Resp. Cell Mol. Biol.* **2:** 553.

Sottrup-Jensen, L. 1989. Alpha-macroglobulins: Structure, shape, and mechanism of proteinase complex formation. *J. Biol. Chem.* **264:** 11539.

Spencer, H. 1977. The pneumoconioses and other occupational lung diseases. In *Pathology of the lung,* p. 371. Pergamon Press, New York.

Sporn, M.B., A.B. Roberts, L.M. Wakefield, and B. deCrombrugghe. 1987. Some recent advances in the chemistry and biology of transforming growth factor-beta. *J. Cell Biol.* **105:** 1039.

Tovey, M.G. 1988. The expression of cytokines in the organs of normal individuals: Role in homeostasis. A review. *J. Biol. Regul. Homeostatic Agents* **2:** 87.

Van Furth, R. and Z.A. Cohn. 1968. The origin and kinetics of mononuclear phagocytes. *J. Exp. Med.* **128:** 415.

Warheit, D.B., L.H. Hill, G. George, and A.R. Brody. 1986. Time course of chemotactic factor generation and the corresponding macrophage response to asbestos inhalation. *Am. Rev. Respir. Dis.* **134:** 128.

Warheit, D.B., G. George, L.H. Hill, R. Snyderman, and A.R. Brody. 1985. Inhaled asbestos activates a complement-dependent chemoattractant for macrophages. *Lab. Invest.* **52:** 505.

Zigmond, S.H. and J.G. Hirsch. 1973. Leukocyte locomotion and chemotaxis. New methods for evaluation, and demonstration of a cell derived chemotactic factor. *J. Exp. Med.* **137:** 387.

Activated Alveolar Macrophages from Individuals with Asbestosis Release Peptide Growth Factors

W.N. Rom

Division of Pulmonary and Critical Care Medicine, Departments of Medicine and Environmental Medicine and Chest Service, Bellevue Hospital, New York University Medical Center, New York, New York

INTRODUCTION

Asbestosis is an interstitial lung disease characterized by thickened alveolar walls and the accumulation of inflammatory cells that are predominantly alveolar macrophages (AMs) but that also include neutrophils and lymphocytes (Jaurand et al. 1980; Craighead and Mossman 1982; Craighead et al. 1982; Gellert et al. 1985; Robinson et al. 1986; Rom et al. 1987). Asbestos fibers are phagocytosed by AMs and in the process become "activated" by changes in their morphology and spontaneous release of mediators including peptide growth factors (Rom et al. 1987; Takemura et al. 1989). These growth factors are chemotactic for mesenchymal cells and stimulate them to proliferate. Growth factors identified in humans with asbestosis include fibronectin, which is a large glycoprotein that acts as a competence growth factor early in the G_1 phase of the fibroblast cell cycle, and AM insulin-like growth factor-I (AMIGF-I), which is a small peptide that acts late in the G_1 phase as a progression growth factor (Rennard et al. 1981; Rom et al. 1987, 1988). Platelet-derived growth factor (PDGF) is a potent mitogenic signal, acting early in the G_1 phase as a competence factor and is considered to provide the majority of growth stimulatory activity released by macrophages (Shimokado et al. 1985; Martinet et al. 1987). PDGF is also known to stimulate a series of genes known as "competence" genes, including c-myc, following attachment to its receptor and before mitogenesis ensues (Kelly et al. 1983; Kelly 1986). The PDGF

B-chain encodes sequences of the c-*sis* proto-oncogene that is activated prior to c-*myc*, providing for hierarchy in the activation process (Dalla Favera et al. 1981; Devare et al. 1983; Doolittle et al. 1983; Robbins et al. 1983; Waterfield et al. 1983; Chiu et al. 1984; Johnsson et al. 1984; Kelly 1986). In this context, asbestosis, a fibrotic interstitial disease with markedly increased risk for cancer when ᴖoupled with smoking, would be a logical disease in which to evaluate PDGF release and expression of the relevant proto-oncogenes in activated AMs.

ASBESTOSIS AND GROWTH FACTORS

In asbestosis, AMs increase in number, have a morphological appearance of activation, and spontaneously release exaggerated amounts of the oxidants, superoxide anion and hydrogen peroxide (Rom et al. 1987; Takemura et al. 1989). Oxidants are toxic to alveolar epithelial cells and fibroblasts, and this burden may contribute to alveolar wall injury in asbestosis (Cantin et al. 1989). AMs from asbestos-exposed individuals also release significantly increased amounts of fibronectin, a large, 220-kD glycoprotein that is chemotactic for fibroblasts, provides an attachment site for cells to the extracellular matrix, and serves as a competence growth factor acting early in the G_1 phase to signal fibroblasts to replicate (Rennard et al. 1981; Rom et al. 1987). In addition to fibronectin, AMs release significantly increased amounts of AM-derived growth factor (AMDGF), an 18–26-kD peptide that acts later in the G_1 phase as a progression growth factor (Rom et al. 1987). These two growth factors act synergistically, signaling fibroblasts to replicate (Bitterman et al. 1983). The AMDGF has been identified to be an AMIGF-I-type molecule similar to tissue-type fibroblast IGF-I by several lines of evidence: AMIGF-I and recombinant IGF-I (rIGF-I) track together on anion-exchange chromatography, an anti-IGF-I monoclonal antibody reduced AMDGF-induced growth activity in serum-free complementation tests in a dose-dependent manner, AMIGF-I and rIGF-I displaced labeled IGF-I from the receptor in a radio-receptor competitive binding assay, and AMIGF-I and rIGF-I both activated the fibroblast IGF-I receptor to phosphorylate a tyrosine-containing artificial substrate (Rom et al. 1988).

ASBESTOSIS AND PDGF

AMs and activated blood monocytes have been shown to express the c-*sis* proto-oncogene, the B-chain of PDGF, and spontaneously release a PDGF-like molecule (Martinet et al. 1986; Mornex et al. 1986). In patients with idiopathic pulmonary fibrosis (IPF), a progressive fibrotic lung disease resulting in death in 1–6 years, exaggerated quantities of this potent competence growth factor were released by AMs (Martinet et al. 1987). Lung epithelial cells and macrophages in the interstitium expressed c-*sis* during in situ hybridization in five patients with IPF (Antoniades et al. 1990). AMs lavaged from IPF patients reveal increased steady-state mRNA levels and transcription rates for PDGF A- and B-chains compared with those of normal controls (Nagaoka et al. 1990). PDGF is a 31-kD peptide that is a chemoattractant for smooth-muscle cells, fibroblasts, neutrophils, and monocytes and is mitogenic for smooth-muscle cells, fibroblasts, and glial cells (Ross et al. 1986). The B-chain of PDGF contains homologous sequences (87%) of v-*sis*; when 3T3 fibroblasts are infected with v-*sis*, they dedifferentiate and exhibit the features of uncontrolled proliferation characteristic of neoplastic cells (Ross et al. 1986; LaRochelle et al. 1990). 3T3 cells transformed with v-*sis* produce the $p^{28\ v\text{-}sis}$ protein analogous to the B-chain of PDGF, which is capable of binding intracellular PDGF receptors and stimulating autocrine growth (LaRochelle et al. 1990). PDGF is contained in the α granules of platelets and is released by platelets in wounds that contribute to mesenchymal cell proliferation in the healing process (Ross et al. 1986). PDGF exists as three dimers: AA, BB, and AB, with BB considered to have the greatest mitogenic activity and circulates complexed with α_2-macroglobulin as a binding protein (Bonner et al. 1989). Evaluation of supernatants from AMs obtained from five individuals with asbestosis and seven controls revealed significantly increased amounts of PDGF chemotactic activity

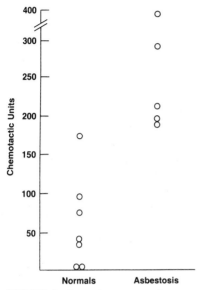

FIGURE 1 Spontaneous release of PDGF chemotactic activity in AM supernatants. Chemotactic activity for smooth-muscle cells was performed with modified Boyden chambers with the lower wells filled with AM supernatants and the upper wells filled with smooth-muscle cells obtained from fetal bovine aorta (Martinet et al. 1987). The numbers of migrating cells were determined by counting cells with a microscope under oil immersion (magnification, 400x) with the slides coded to blind the reader, and the chemotactic activity was expressed in chemotactic units released per 10^6 AM/24 hr. AMs lavaged from five nonsmoking individuals with asbestosis (age in yr, mean 58 ± 2 S.E. and asbestos exposure mean, 38 ± 3 S.E.) spontaneously released more PDGF than normal controls (p <0.05). All of the asbestos workers had interstitial fibrosis and pleural plaques on their chest X-rays and a restrictive pattern of pulmonary function.

(Fig. 1, asbestos-exposed 255 ± 46 units vs. control 60 ± 23 units, p <0.05).

Previous experiments have demonstrated that AM chemotactic activity for smooth-muscle cells was PDGF (Martinet et al. 1986; Mornex et al. 1986). First, PDGF (5 μg/ml) attracted the same number of smooth-muscle cells as unfractionated AM supernatant in the chemotaxis assay (Martinet et al. 1987). Second, the activity was reduced by $85 \pm 5\%$ by anti-PDGF antibody, and human fetal lung fibroblast proliferation was inhibited in a serum-free complementation assay by the same antibody (Martinet et al. 1987). Third, AM supernatant was shown to compete with ^{125}I-labeled PDGF for binding to the PDGF receptor on fibroblasts in a dose-dependent manner similar to that of purified PDGF (Mornex et al. 1986). Fourth, a radioimmunoassay using anti-PDGF antibody found AM supernatants contain a molecule that is antigenically similar to that of PDGF (Martinet et al. 1987). Finally, PDGF and the AM chemotactic activity coeluted as a single peak at 31 kD, using molecular sieve chromatography (Mornex et al. 1986; Martinet et al. 1987).

AM from asbestosis are activated and not only spontaneously release significantly increased amounts of PDGF compared with that of controls, but they also express a 4.2-kb mRNA transcript for the c-*sis* gene that is similar to what has been reported previously for other interstitial lung diseases: sarcoidosis, histiocytosis X, and idiopathic pulmonary fibrosis (Mornex et al. 1986).

ASBESTOSIS AND CANCER

Asbestosis is associated with an increased risk for lung cancer and mesothelioma, as well as other malignancies. The mortality experience of 17,800 United States and Canadian asbestos insulation workers has been studied prospectively from January 1, 1967, with death certificates and "best evidence" including biopsy, radiography, and autopsy records to correct for death certificate misclassification among the exposed. The standardized mortality ratio for all causes of death was 146 with a threefold excess of all cancer deaths that was primarily the following: lung cancer with 1166 deaths observed and 267 deaths expected (ratio 4.36); 457 mesothelioma deaths observed; 189 gastrointestinal cancer deaths observed with 135 deaths expected (ratio 1.4, which was highest for esophagus); 18 laryngeal cancer deaths observed with 10.5 deaths expected (ratio 1.71); 48 oral cavity cancer deaths observed with 22 deaths expected (ratio 2.2); and increased kidney cancer (Selikoff et al. 1979). The multiplicative effect of asbestos exposure and smoking for lung cancer was reported by Selikoff et al. (1968). In a review of the study of 544 deaths due to bronchogenic carcinoma in United States and Canadian asbestos insulation workers, only 4 were nonsmokers of 471 for whom smoking histories were available (Suzuki and Selikoff 1986). Histologic fibrosis was found in lung tissue in 355 of 356 available samples, and asbestos bodies were observed in 96.6% of the sample (Suzuki and Selikoff 1986).

ASBESTOSIS AND ONCOGENES

Because individuals with >20 years of occupational exposure to asbestos are at risk for alveolitis, interstitial pulmonary fibrosis, and malignancy, it seemed reasonable to evaluate AMs, which are cells that are easily obtainable and are a major participant in the inflammatory and fibrotic processes for proto-oncogene expression (Heldin and Westermark 1984). AMs lavaged from individuals with asbestosis expressed a 2.3-kb mRNA for the c-*myc* proto-oncogene (Fig. 2). The cytotrophoblast of the developing human placenta expresses *myc* and *sis* mRNAs and releases and responds to PDGF in an autocrine manner (Goustin et al. 1985). The c-*myc* gene is the cellular homolog of the transforming determinant carried by the avian myelocytomatosis virus (Cole 1986). It is expressed in the human promyelocytic leukemia cell line, HL-60, and in Burkitt's lymphoma (Gowda et al. 1986; Kelly 1986). The c-*myc* gene is translocated adjacent to the immunoglobulin heavy-chain locus, resulting in enhanced expression (Kelly 1986). The c-*myc* protein is found in the nucleus and binds to DNA sequences thought to regulate the transcription of genes whose products ultimately cause cellular division (Perrson and Leder 1984). Leukemic cells grown in vitro are unable to suppress the transcription of c-*myc* (Gowda et al. 1986). The c-*myc* gene is also expressed in the early competence stage of the cell cycle and is induced by PDGF in BALB/c-3T3 cells (~40-fold in 3 hr), B lymphocytes with lipopolysaccharide, and T lymphocytes after activation with concanavalin A (Kelly et al. 1983; Kelly 1986). In contrast, c-*myc* mRNA is not induced following EGF or insulin treatment or IGF-I treatment of quiescent BALB/c-3T3 cells, but EGF can induce c-*myc* in NIH-3T3 cells or in a cell that proliferatively responds to EGF binding

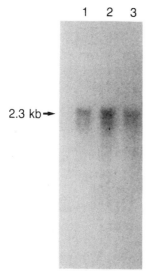

FIGURE 2 Expression of 2.3-kb mRNA transcript after hybridization with c-*myc* exon III cDNA probe using Northern blot analysis. The *ClaI* exon III human c-*myc* probe was kindly provided by Dr. Kathleen Kelly of the National Cancer Institute (Battey et al. 1983). All three lanes have 10 µg of total RNA extracted from AMs from three individuals with asbestosis.

(Kelly et al. 1983; Müller et al. 1984; Kelly and Siebenlist 1985; Kelly 1986). Phorbol-12-myristate-13-acetate activates protein kinase C and enhances c-*myc* expression analogous to PDGF, but neither protein kinase C nor c-*myc* activation accounts for the mitogenic action of PDGF, indicating other essential pathways (Coughlin et al. 1985).

Kelly et al. (1984) has postulated that the protein encoded by an oncogene (e.g., c-*sis*), inducing the expression of another oncogene (c-*myc*), is an example of how oncogenes could interact in hierarchies to stimulate malignant growth. In asbestosis, the stimulus for AM activation (asbestos) is persistent, which may result in continuous stimulation of AM proto-oncogenes (e.g., c-*sis* and c-*myc*) with exaggerated release of growth signals leading to enhanced mesenchymal cell and possibly other cell proliferation in a paracrine manner. In addition, the presence of these proto-oncogenes in the inflammatory milieu of the alveolar spaces may provide opportunity for DNA bound to fibers to be transfected into neighboring epithelial cells and may play a role in cellular transformation (Appel et al. 1988). Asbestos fibers might cause a mutation in a proto-oncogene altering transcription or release of tumor suppressor capability (Jackson et al. 1987). The *myc* family of oncogenes has been reported previously to be amplified in lung cancer (Nau et al. 1985; Johnson et al. 1987; Viallet and Minna 1990). This preliminary study raises the question of whether AMs are able to up-regulate c-*myc* when in the activated state after asbestos exposure or whether expression is constitutive. These preliminary results suggest that activated AM recovered by bronchoalveolar lavage from individuals with asbestosis spontaneously express c-*myc* and c-*sis* and release exaggerated amounts of PDGF, which is a mediator that likely serves a function for chemotaxis and mitogenesis of lung mesenchymal cells.

ACKNOWLEDGMENTS

The author thanks Y. Martinet for performing the chemotaxis assays, K. Kelly for the c-*myc* cDNA probe, the Pulmonary Branch of the National Heart, Lung, and Blood Institute for assistance, and Kathleen Neville for typing the manuscript.

REFERENCES

Antoniades, H.N., M.A. Bravo, R.E. Avila, T. Galanopoulos, J. Neville-Golden, M. Maxwell, and M. Selman. 1990. Platelet-derived growth factor in idiopathic pulmonary fibrosis. *J. Clin. Invest.* **86:** 1055.

Appel, J.D., T.M. Fasy, D.S. Kohtz, J.D. Kohtz, and E.M. Johnson. 1988. Asbestos fibers mediate transformation of monkey cells by exogenous plasmid DNA. *Proc. Natl. Acad. Sci.* **85:** 7670.

Battey, J., C. Moulding, R. Taub, W. Murphy, T. Stewart, H. Potter, G. Lenoir, and P. Leder. 1983. The human c-*myc* oncogene: Structural consequences of translocation into the IgH locus in Burkitt lymphoma. *Cell* **34:** 779.

Bitterman, P.B., S.I. Rennard, S. Adelberg, and R.G. Crystal. 1983. Role of fibronectin as a growth factor for fibroblasts. *J. Cell Biol.* **97:** 1925.

Bonner, J.C., M. Hoffman, and A.R. Brody. 1989. Alpha-macroglobulin secreted by alveolar macrophages serves as a binding protein for a macrophage-derived homologue of platelet-derived growth factor. *Am. J. Respir. Cell Mol. Biol.* **1:** 171.

Cantin, A.M., S.L. North, G.A. Fells, R.C. Hubbard, and R.G. Crystal. 1989. Oxidant-mediated epithelial cell injury in idiopathic pulmonary fibrosis. *J. Clin. Invest.* **79:** 1665.

Chiu, I.-M., E.P. Reddy, D. Givol, K.C. Robbins, S.R. Tronick, and S.A. Aaronson. 1984. Nucleotide sequence analysis identifies the human c-*sis* proto-oncogene as a structural gene for platelet-derived growth factor. *Cell* **37:** 123.

Cole, M. 1986. The *myc* oncogene: Its role in transformation and differentiation. *Annu. Rev. Genet.* **20:** 361.

Coughlin, S.R., W.M.F. Lee, P.W. Williams, G.M. Giels, and L.T. Williams. 1985. c-*myc* gene expression is stimulated by agents that activate protein kinase C and does not account for the mitogenic effect of PDGF. *Cell* **43:** 243.

Craighead, J.E. and B.T. Mossman. 1982. The pathogenesis of asbestos-associated diseases. *N. Engl. J. Med.* **306:** 1446.

Craighead, J.E., J.L. Abraham, A. Churg, F.H.Y. Green, J. Kleinerman, P.C. Pratt, T.A. Seemayer, V. Vallyathan, and H. Weill. 1982. The pathology of asbestos-associated diseases of the lungs and pleural cavities: Diagnostic criteria and proposed grading schema. *Arch. Pathol. Lab. Med.* **106:** 544.

Dalla Favera, R., E.P. Gelmann, R.C. Gallo, and F. Wong-Staal. 1981. A human *onc* gene homologous to the transforming gene (v-*sis*) of simian sarcoma virus. *Nature* **292:** 31.

Devare, S.G., E.P. Reddy, J.D. Law, K.C. Robbins, and S.A. Aaronson. 1983. Nucleotide sequence of the simian sarcoma virus genome: Demonstration that its acquired cellular sequences encode the transforming gene product p28^{sis}. *Proc. Natl. Acad. Sci.* **80:** 731.

Doolittle, R.F., M.W. Hunkapiller, L.E. Hood, S.G. Devare, K.C. Robbins, S.A. Aaronson, and H.N. Antoniades. 1983. Simian sarcoma virus *onc* gene, v-*sis*, is derived from the gene (or genes) encoding a platelet-derived growth factor. *Science* **221:** 275.

Gellert, A.R., M.G. Macey, S. Uthayakumar, A.C. Newland, and R.M. Rudd. 1985. Lymphocyte subpopulations in bronchoalveolar lavage fluid in asbestos workers. *Am. Rev. Respir. Dis.* **132:** 824.

Goustin, A.S., C. Betsholtz, S. Pfeifer-Ohlsson, H. Persson, J. Rydnert, M. Bywater, G. Holmgren, C.-H. Heldin, B. Westermark, and R. Ohlsson. 1985. Coexpression of the *sis* and *myc* proto-oncogenes in developing human placenta suggests autocrine control of trophoblast growth. *Cell* **41:** 301.

Gowda, S.D., R.D. Koler, and G.C. Bagby, Jr. 1986. Regulation of c-*myc* expression during growth and differentiation of normal and leukemic human myeloid progenitor cells. *J. Clin. Invest.* **77:** 271.

Heldin, C.-H. and B. Westermark. 1984. Growth factors: Mechanism of action and relation to oncogenes. *Cell* **37:** 9.

Jackson, J.H., I.U. Schraufstatter, P.A. Hyslop, K. Vosbeck, R. Sauer-heber, S.A. Weitsman, and C.G. Cochrane. 1987. Role of oxidants in DNA damage. Hydroxyl radical mediates the synergistic DNA damaging effects of asbestos and cigarette smoke. *J. Clin. Invest.* **80:** 1090.

Jaurand, M.C., A. Gaudichet, K. Atassi, P. Sébastien, and J. Bignon. 1980. Relationship between the number of asbestos fibres and the cellular and enzymatic content of bronchoalveolar fluid in asbestos exposed subjects. *Bull. Europ. Physiopathol. Respir.* **16:** 595.

Johnson, B.E., D.C. Ihde, R.W. Makuch, A.F. Gazdar, D.N. Carney, H. Ole, E. Russell, M.M. Nau, and J.D. Minna. 1987. *Myc* family oncogene amplification in tumor cell lines established from small cell lung cancer patients and its relationship to clinical status and course. *J. Clin. Invest.* **79:** 1629.

Johnsson, A., C.-H. Heldin, A. Wasteson, B. Westermark, T.F. Deuel, J.S. Huang, P.H. Seeburg, A. Gray, A. Ullrich, G. Scrace, P. Stroobant, and M.D. Waterfield. 1984. The c-*sis* gene encodes a precursor of the B chain of platelet-derived growth factor. *EMBO J.* **3:** 921.

Kelly, K. 1986. The regulation and expression of c-*myc* in normal malignant cells. *Annu. Rev. Immunol.* **4:** 317.

Kelly, K. and U. Siebenlist. 1985. The role of c-*myc* in the proliferation of normal and neoplastic cells. *J. Clin. Immunol.* **5:** 65.

Kelly, K., B.H. Cochran, C.D. Stiles, and P. Leder. 1983. Cell-specific regulation of the c-*myc* gene by lymphocyte mitogens and platelet-derived growth factor. *Cell* **35:** 603.

―――. 1984. The regulation of c-*myc* by growth signals. *Curr. Top. Microbiol. Immunol.* **113:** 117.

LaRochelle, W.J., N. Giese, M. May-Siroff, K.C. Robbins, and S.A. Aaronson. 1990. Molecular localization of the transforming and secretory properties of PDGF A and PDGF B. *Science* **248:** 1541.

Martinet, Y., W.N. Rom, G.R. Grotendorst, G.R. Martin, R.G. Crystal. 1987. Exaggerated spontaneous release of platelet-derived growth factor by alveolar macrophages from patients with idiopathic pulmonary fibrosis. *N. Engl. J. Med.* **317:** 202.

Martinet, Y., P.B. Bitterman, J.-F. Mornex, G.R. Grotendorst, G.R. Martin, and R.G. Crystal. 1986. Activated human monocytes express the c-*sis* proto-oncogene and release a mediator showing PDGF-like activity. *Nature* **319:** 158.

Mornex, J.-F., Y. Martinet, K. Yamauchi, P.B. Bitterman, G.R. Grotendorst, A. Chytil-Weir, G.R. Martin, and R.G. Crystal. 1986. Spontaneous expression of c-*sis* gene and release of platelet-derived growth factor-like molecule by human alveolar macrophages. *J. Clin. Invest.* **78:** 61.

Müller, R., R. Bravo, J. Burckhardt, and T. Curran. 1984. Induction of c-*fos* gene and protein by growth factors precedes activation by c-*myc*. *Nature* **312:** 317.

Nagaoka, I., B.C. Trapnell, and R.G. Crystal. 1990. Upregulation of platelet-derived growth factor-A and -B gene expression in alveolar macrophages of individuals with idiopathic pulmonary fibrosis. *J. Clin. Invest.* **85:** 2023.

Nau, M.M., B.J. Brooks, J. Battey, E. Sausville, A.F. Gazdar, I.R. Kirsch, O.W. McBride, V. Bertness, G.F. Hollis, and J.D. Minna. 1985. L-*myc*, a new *myc*-related gene amplified and expressed in human small cell lung cancer. *Nature* **318:** 69.

Perrson, H. and P. Leder. 1984. Nuclear localization and DNA binding properties of a protein expressed by human c-*myc* oncogene. *Science* **225:** 718.

Rennard, S.I., G.W. Hunninghake, P.B. Bitterman, and R.G. Crystal. 1981. Production of fibronectin by the human alveolar macrophage: Mechanism for the recruitment of fibroblasts to sites of tissue injury in interstitial lung diseases. *Proc. Natl. Acad. Sci.* **78:** 7147.

Robbins, K.C., H.N. Antoniades, S.G. Devare, M.W. Hunkapiller, S.A. Aaronson. 1983. Structural and immunological similarities between simian sarcoma virus gene product(s) and human platelet-derived growth factor. *Nature* **305:** 605.

Robinson, B.W.S., A.H. Rose, A. James, D. Whitaker, and A.W. Musk. 1986. Alveolitis of pulmonary asbestosis. Bronchoalveolar lavage studies in crocidolite- and chrysotile-exposed individuals. *Chest* **90:** 396.

Rom, W.N., P.B. Bitterman, S.I. Rennard, A. Cantin, and R.G. Crystal. 1987. Characterization of the lower respiratory tract inflammation of non-smoking individuals with interstitial lung disease associated with chronic inhalation of inorganic dusts. *Am. Rev. Respir. Dis.* **136:** 1429.

Rom, W.N., P. Basset, G.A. Fells, T. Nukiwa, B.C. Trapnell, and R.G. Crystal. 1988. Alveolar macrophages release in insulin-like growth factor I-type molecule. *J. Clin. Invest.* **82:** 1685.

Ross, R., E.W. Raines, D.F. Bowen-Pope. 1986. The biology of platelet-derived growth factor. *Cell* **46:** 155.

Selikoff, I.J., E.C. Hammond, and J. Churg. 1968. Asbestos exposure: Smoking, and neoplasia. *J. Am. Med. Assoc.* **204:** 106.

Selikoff, I.J., E.C. Hammond, and H. Seidman. 1979. Mortality experience of insulation workers in the United States and Canada, 1943–1976. *Ann. N.Y. Acad. Sci.* **330:** 91.

Shimokado, K., E.W. Raines, D.K. Madtes, T.B. Barrett, E.P. Benditt, and R. Ross. 1985. A significant part of macrophage-derived growth factor consists of at least two forms of PDGF. *Cell* **43:** 277.

Suzuki, Y. and I.J. Selikoff. 1986. Pathology of lung cancer among asbestos insulation workers. *Fed. Proc.* **45:** 744A.

Takemura, T., W.N. Rom, V.J. Ferrans, and R.G. Crystal. 1989. Morphological characterization of alveolar macrophages from individuals with occupational exposure to inorganic particles. *Am. Rev.*

Respir. Dis. **140:** 1674.

Viallet, J. and J.D. Minna. 1990. Dominant oncogenes and tumor suppressor genes in the pathogenesis of lung cancer. *Am. J. Respir. Cell Mol. Biol.* **2:** 225.

Waterfield, M.D., G.T. Scrace, N. Whittle, P. Stroobant, A. Johnsson, A. Wasteson, B. Westermark, C.-H. Heldin, J.S. Huang, and T.F. Deuel. 1983. Platelet-derived growth factor is structurally related to the putative transforming protein p28^{sis} of simian sarcoma virus. *Nature* **304:** 35.

Studies on Human Mesothelial Cells: Effects of Growth Factors and Asbesti-form Fibers

J.F. Lechner, B.I. Gerwin, R.R. Reddel,[1] E.W. Gabrielson,[2] A. Van der Meeren, K. Linnainmaa,[3] A.N.A. Somers,[4] and C.C. Harris

Laboratory of Human Carcinogenesis, Division of Cancer Etiology, National Cancer Institute, National Institutes of Health, Bethesda, Maryland 20892

INTRODUCTION

Pleural mesothelioma is caused by asbesti-form fibers (Craighead and Mossman 1982). The biological properties of the putative target cell of this human disease, the mesothelial cell, are different from other types of lung epithelial cells. Specifically, these cells have a plastic cytoskeleton (Wu et al. 1982; Connell and Rheinwald 1983; LaRocca and Rheinwald 1985) and are especially sensitive to the cytotoxic effects of asbestos in vitro (Lechner et al. 1983, 1985a). However, the mechanisms by which fibers bring about neoplastic transformation of mesothelial cells is unclear. Presumably, this mechanism relates to the clastogenic activity of these fibers (Hesterberg and Barrett 1985; Lechner et al. 1985a,b; Wang et al. 1987). Although fibers do not directly induce oxyradical production by human mesothelial cells (Gabrielson et al. 1988b), such radicals might be generated by fiber activation of macrophages (Mossman and Marsh 1989).

GROWTH REQUIREMENTS OF NORMAL HUMAN MESOTHELIAL CELLS

Sustained Replication versus a Single Round of DNA Synthesis

To study the fiber-mesothelial cell interaction, it was critical to investigate the cell biology of normal mesothelial cells of ani-

Present addresses: [1]Children's Medical Research Foundation, Camperdown, New South Wales 2050, Australia; [2]Francis Scott Key Medical Center, Baltimore, MD 21224; [3]Institute of Occupational Health, SF-00250 Helsinki, Finland; [4]Dept. of Epithelial Biology, Paterson Institute for Cancer Research, Manchester, England.

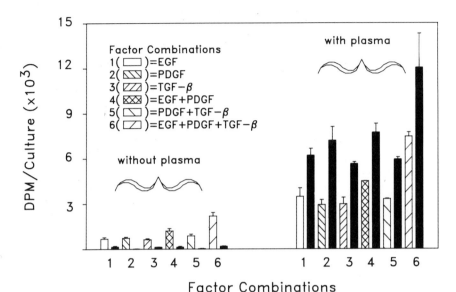

FIGURE 1 Effects of growth factors on first round and sustained DNA synthesis. (Open boxes) First-round growth rates between 18 and 32 hr of incubation after addition of growth factor to quiescent cultures; (solid symbols) sustained growth rates measured between 66 and 90 hr after addition of the growth factor.

mal and especially human origin. Rheinwald and co-workers (Wu et al. 1982; Lechner et al. 1983) determined that normal human mesothelial (NHM) cells require a rich nutrient medium supplemented with epidermal growth factor (EGF), hydrocortisone, insulin, and fetal bovine serum (FBS) for growth. Subsequently, we found that platelet-derived growth factor (PDGF, [A/B heterodimer]) and transforming growth factor-β (TGF-β_1) are mitogenic for NHM cells (Gabrielson et al. 1988a). In addition, these two factors can act in concert, both with EGF and/or with each other, to stimulate greater growth rates. However, even in a medium containing both EGF and PDGF or TGF-β_1, the cells fail to undergo more than one round of DNA synthesis unless FBS or plasma is also present (Fig. 1).

Chemically denatured serum (CDS) (van Zoelen et al. 1985, 1986) has been reported as a comitogen for supporting anchorage-independent growth of transformed cells. CDS is thought to have no active peptide growth factors because they are denatured by dithiothreitol (DTT) and 5-iodoacetamide (5-IA) treatments. CDS did support sustained growth of NHM cells when added to medium containing EGF (LaVeck et al. 1988). On the other hand, replacement of FBS with CDS did not alter the differential growth vigor among the individual NHM cell cultures (see below). Van Zoelen et al. (1985, 1986) attributed the comitogenic activity of CDS to fibronectin (fn), which is not inactivated by the DTT/5-IA. Nevertheless, we found that FN could not substitute for plasma as a comitogen for NHM cells. Polyacrylamide gel electrophoresis of CDS revealed three major bands between 50 and 80 kD and two larger bands estimated to be between 120 and 170 kD in CDS that were comigratory with commercial high-density lipoproteins (HDL). Therefore, HDL was purified from CDS and assayed. As can be seen (Fig. 2), the extraction procedure increased the specific activity and the mitogenic activity equally, suggesting that the majority of the comitogenic activity of CDS for human mesothelial cells is associated with HDL. Because considerable donor variation in growth response to FBS had been noted, the experiments were repeated with cells obtained from eight different donors using media containing CDS. As can be seen (Fig. 3), all supported sustained growth, although no donors' cells were uniformly responsive to all the mitogens.

Interindividual Variability among Normal Human Mesothelial Cells

It was also of interest that, from donor to donor, there was considerable variation in growth vigor of NHM cells in culture. Secondary cultures from 57 donors expressed (Fig. 4) a continuum of growth rates (Lechner et al. 1989). Of the cultures that exemplified the complete range of growth vigor, 14 were subcultured and reassayed. The incorporated [^{3}H]thymidine culture was not significantly different from that observed for the previous passage. Thus, growth vigor is not a function of the population doubling level of the culture but is due to inherent interindividual variation. We also assessed other mitogens: aqueous bovine pituitary extract (BPE), cholera toxin (CT), interleukin-1 (IL-1), interleukin-2 (IL-2), basic fibroblast

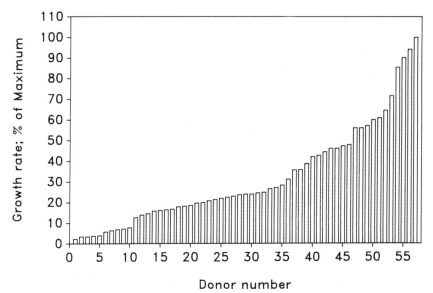

FIGURE 2 Variation if growth rate of secondary NHM cell cultures form 57 individuals.

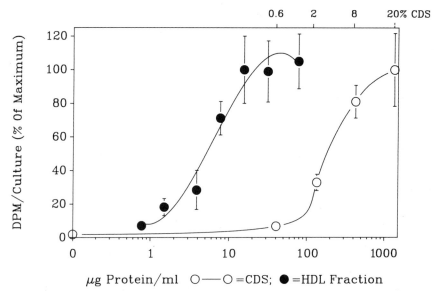

FIGURE 3 Mitogenicity of CDS and HDL extracted therefrom. The purification procedure increased the specific activity of the HDL fraction 200-fold.

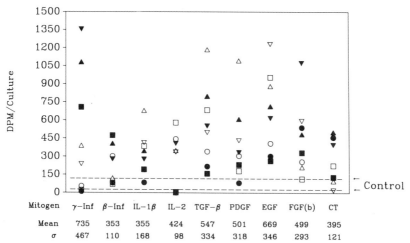

Mitogen	γ-Inf	β-Inf	IL-1β	IL-2	TGF-β	PDGF	EGF	FGF(b)	CT
Mean	735	353	355	424	547	501	669	499	395
σ	467	110	168	98	334	318	346	293	121

FIGURE 4 Relative growth stimulation of NHM cells developed from eight donors by peptide mitogens. (Dashed lines) Control range (no mitogen) values.

growth factor (bFGF), interleukin-3 (IL-3), triio-dothyronine (T_3), glucagon, β human chorionic gonadotropin, bombesin, α-interferon, β-interferon (INF-β), γ-interferon (INF-γ); epinephrine, retinoic acid, fatty acids solution (palmitic, stearic, palmitoleic, oleic, linoleic, and linolenic [Laemmli 1970]), and insulin-like growth factor-1. None of these supported sustained growth of NHM cells. However, like EGF, TGF-β and PDGF, INF-β, BPE, CT, bFGF, IL-1, IL-2, and INF-γ, also induced the cells to synthesize DNA for one cell cycle.

It is known that activated macrophages elaborate numerous mitogens (Hartmann et al. 1984; Assoian et al. 1987; Nathan 1987; Kumar et al. 1988). Thus, although no correlation was found between the clinical diagnosis of the donor and response to specific growth factor, each individual culture of NHM cells could have been previously "imprinted" in vivo to respond to a unique battery of mitogens that had been elaborated into the pleural fluid by macrophages in response to clinical or subclinical infections, and so forth. To test this possibility, NHM cells from six donors were initially incubated in serum-containing growth medium for one passage. Each donor's cells were then subcultured and incubated in five dif-

TABLE 1 THE EFFECT OF PREINCUBATION WITH A SINGLE FACTOR OF THE SUBSEQUENT RESPONSE TO A PANEL OF FACTORS

Preincubation factor	Mitogenic response				
	EGF	INF-γ	IL-1β	PDGF	bFGF
None	100	40	4	98	14
EGF	104	39	6	93	11
INF-γ	84	39	3	80	10
IL-1β	88	34	5	79	9
PDGF	99	38	11	87	11
bFGF	73	32	6	85	15

A culture on NHM cells was established in FBS-containing medium. It was then subcultured, the growth rate was measured in media containing CDS and one of the listed factors, and the growth rates were recorded. Sister cultures from each of the above CDS/factor media were then dissociated, and the growth rates were reassayed using all of the CDS/factor media. The growth rates are stated relative to the none/EGF value.

ferent media (CDS/EGF, CDS/FGF, CDS/PDGF, CDS/IL-1, CDS/INF-γ). The growth rates were then measured, and the cells were reinoculated into all of the above listed five media. Thus, for each donor, growth was first measured postincubation in FBS-containing medium in five different CDS/factor media. Subsequently, each culture was reassayed. If the cells imprint, best growth should be obtained in the medium of the previous passage. A typical result is shown in Table 1, the data for the others were comparable (Lechner et al. 1989). As can be seen, imprinting did not occur. Instead, the variation is inherent in the cell strain.

GROWTH FACTOR PRODUCTION BY NORMAL MESOTHELIAL CELLS AND MESOTHELIOMAS

Because NHM cells respond to the mitogenic signals of several growth factors, many of which are released by activated macrophages, one scenario for promotion of asbesti-form-fiber-initiated mesothelial cells is that the growth factor environment causes them to evolve into a large population for subsequent genetic insults, such as macrophage-mediated oxidative damage. Expansion of an asbestos-initiated mesothelial cell as a response to these macrophage-released factors would be a function of that cell's inherent reaction to the specific growth factor. Thus, the interindividual variation in growth control that we have described for NHM cells could be important in determining the probability that an exposed individual would develop mesothelioma. In addition, acquired production of autocrine growth factors is thought to be a pivotal step in the evolution of some tumors (Sporn and Todaro 1980).

Because growth of NHM cells can be stimulated by numerous mitogens, they provide a large target for dysregulated genes that could result in autocrine growth factor production. To assess this possibility, we assayed conditioned media from numerous mesothelioma cell cultures for their ability to promote growth of NHM cells (Gerwin et al. 1987, 1990). Several of these were growth stimulatory, and one (HUT28) contained PDGF-like activity. Therefore, mesothelioma and NHM cells were assessed for PDGF A-chain and B-chain messages. All mesothelioma cell lines tested overexpressed A-chain message, and some lines also expressed B-chain mRNA (Gerwin et al. 1987). Only a low level of A-chain mRNA was detected in the NHM cells.

To test the role of PDGF A-chain overproduction in the pathogenesis of mesothelioma, DNA constructs containing this gene have been recently introduced into SV40 T-antigen gene "immortalized" nontumorigenic (MeT-5A; [Ke et al. 1989]) human mesothelial cells (Van der Meeren et al. 1990). Transfectants were compared with parental and MeT-5A vector control cultures for decreased generation time, increased colony-forming efficiency, and acquisition of the ability to replicate in the absence of FBS and/or growth factors. These changes were quantitatively greater in the A-chain recipient cells. In addition, the A-chain recipient cells were tumorigenic with a mean latency of 7.0 ± 4.9 weeks, whereas the *neo* cultures have remained nontumorigenic. Therefore, these preliminary results indicate that overexpression of PDGF A-chain may be important in the development of some mesotheliomas.

INTERACTIONS OF HUMAN MESOTHELIAL CELLS WITH FIBERS

Examination of Cytoskeletal Effects

The reason for the unique sensitivity of mesothelial cells to the cytotoxic effects of asbesti-form fibers is unknown. Likewise, there is no explanation for the fact that mesothelial cells are more easily transformed than are their airway counterparts (Wagner et al. 1980) by exposure to these fibers, even though fibers encounter the mesothelial cells after passing through the airway. We have suggested that these properties stem from the unique plasticity of the mesothelial cytoskeleton (Lechner et al. 1985a,b). Furthermore, potentially, the responses of cells with keratin intermediate filaments to asbesti-form fibers could be quantitatively different from their vimentin-expressing counterparts. Therefore, we tested whether growth medium containing CDS and either EGF, bFGF, IL-1_β, INF-γ, or PDGF (A/B heterodimer) controlled the expression of polymerized keratin and vimentin similarly (LaVeck et al. 1988). Vimentin microtubules were observed in replicating cells in all media. On the other hand, more than 90% of the cells exhibited polymerized cytokeratin fibers (cytokeratin types 7, 8, 18, and 19) when confluent, even when incubated for 4 days in medium containing any of the above-listed factors. In contrast, nonconfluent cultures showed primarily punctate cytokeratin staining. Thus, direct determinations of cytoskeleton type versus cytotoxic response to fibers is not possible.

The effect of Union International Contre le Cancer standard reference amosite asbestos on the distribution of keratin and vimentin intermediate filaments and cytotubulin in NHM cells is also being investigated. In preliminary experiments, there appears to be no significant difference in the appearance of the cytoskeletons of untreated and amosite-treated cells. Occasionally, larger fibers surrounded by an aura of fluorescence can be detected in the cytoskeletons of treated cells. This fluorescence may represent the binding of individual filament subunits or the filaments themselves to the asbestos fiber. However, it is also possible that this observation is an artifact of the fixation and staining process. If the increase in fluorescence is the result of an interaction between the filaments and the asbestos, clearly the effect is only within a local area of the cell cytoskeleton. It is unlikely that such a local effect on the keratin and vimentin intermediate filaments or on the cytoplasmic microtubules is responsible for the observed structural and numerical chromosome aberrations observed in mesothelial cells after exposure to asbestos fibers.

Comparative Studies of Fiber Effects on Mesothelial or Fibroblastic Cell Mitotic Fidelity

Since it has been established that the fibers quickly become perinuclear (Lechner et al. 1985b), it remains possible that asbestos acts directly on the microtubules that constitute the nuclear spindle and interfere with the spindle formation and/or function. Preliminary investigations of fiber interactions during mitosis are being conducted using the SV40 T-antigen gene immortalized MeT-5A cells. These cells are near diploid (Ke et al. 1989). In addition, they have the typical NHM plastic cytoskeleton, they are equally sensitive to the cytotoxic effects of asbesti-form fibers, and they exhibit a high mitotic rate (Ke et al. 1989). Some preliminary observations can be reported. First, particulates do not disturb division in mesothelial cells. Second, the mitotic fidelity measured for mesothelial cells is less than for fibroblastic cells (Table 2); this tendency to develop aneuploidy and chromosomal aberrations has been noted previously (Linnainmaa et al. 1986 and unpubl.). Third, amosite induces binucleation in both cell types, but the effective dose is more than tenfold higher for fibroblasts than for mesothelial cells (Fig. 5). Fourth, amosite disrupts the fidelity of spindle formation in both fibroblastic and mesothelial cells. In fibroblasts (Table 3), this fiber primarily causes scattered chromatin, but high incidences of chromatin masses and chromosome clusters are also found. In addition, mitotic aberrations, most often in the form of multipolar metaphases, are seen.

The effects on the mesothelial cells were different (Table 4). At the first mitosis, the only significant effects were chromosomal abnormalities, most notably chromosome clustering, which is a mitotic phenotype that is considered to be a very sensitive indicator of spindle damage and subsequent aneuploidy in daughter cells (Parry et al. 1982, 1984; Parry 1985). The effects persisted, and one generation later, mitotic aberrations, specifically multipolar metaphases, were seen (Table 4). In such cells, the disjunction and segregation of the chromosomes at anaphase and telophase would be irregular, resulting in the formation of grossly aneuploid daughter cells. Therefore, on the basis of these preliminary results, it is obvious that am-

TABLE 2 *INDUCTION OF CHROMOSOMAL ABERRATIONS BY AMOSITE ASBESTOS*

Cell type	Threshold dose ($\mu g/cm^2$)	Types of damage
Mesothelial	0.07–0.14	chromatid breaks and gaps; chromosome breaks and gaps; dicentrics
Fibroblastic	2.7–6.7	chromatid breaks and gaps; chromosome breaks

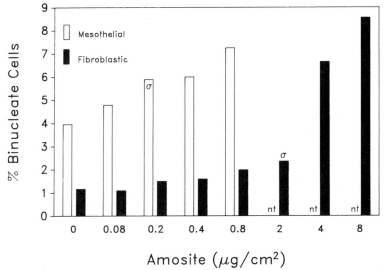

FIGURE 5 Induction of binucleate cells by amosite exposure.

TABLE 3 *FIDELITY OF MITOSIS OF HUMAN FIBROBLASTIC CELLS EXPOSED TO AMOSITE*

Condition	MI[1]	Aberrations[1]				Abnormalities[1]			
		%	D_M	$L_{A/T}$	MP	%	CM	SC	CC
Control	3.2	2.7	2.4	–	0.3	–	0	–	–
With amosite	2.3	6.0	3.0	–	3.0	4.5	0.5	3.0	1.0

[1](MI) Mitotic index; (D_M) chromosome dislocated from mitotic plate; ($L_{A/T}$) lagging chromosomes at anaphase and metaphase; (MP) multipolar metaphase; (CM) chromatin mass; (SC) scattered chromosomes; (CC) chromosome clusters.

TABLE 4 FIDELITY OF MITOSIS OF HUMAN MESOTHELIAL CELLS EXPOSED TO ASBESTOS

Condition	MI[1]	Aberrations[1]				Abnormalities[1]			
		%	D_M	$L_{A/T}$	MP	%	CM	SC	CC
Control	4.9	6.6	3.1	1.2	2.3	3.5	–	0.8	2.7
With amosite (1st mitosis)	5.8	9.2	4.2	2.0	3.0	9.6	0.5	2.6	6.5
With amosite (2nd mitosis)	4.9	11.3	4.0	0.4	6.9	7.2	0.9	0.9	5.0

[1](MI) Mitotic index; (D_M) chromosome dislocated from mitotic plate; $(L_{A/T})$ lagging chromosomes at anaphase and metaphase; (MP) multipolar metaphase; (CM) chromatin mass; (SC) scattered chromosomes; (CC) chromosome clusters.

osite asbestos fibers have the ability to disturb the fidelity of both the first and the second division of MeT-5A cells and hence to induce aneuploid daughter cells. We reported previously (Lechner et al. 1985b) that human mesothelial cells are as much as 20-times more sensitive than bronchial fibroblasts to the effects of amosite fibers. These results cannot be explained by a more active uptake of the fibers in these cells, since quantitative analysis has revealed that both cell types ingest fibers to the same extent (E. Gabrielson, unpubl.).

Code 100 glass fibers also disturb the fidelity of mesothelial cell division and induce aneuploidy (Table 5). Our preliminary results suggest, however, that this kind of fiber works through a different mechanism. Specifically, abnormalities in the form of chromatin masses predominate, and the most common form of mitotic aberration is dislocated chromosomes. In addition, the majority of metaphases observed usually had more than one chromosome dislocated from the spindle at metaphase. This type of effect may be indicative of centromere/kinetochore damage and/or irregular spindle function.

Our preliminary studies differ from those of previous reports (Hesterberg and Barrett 1985; Lechner et al. 1985a) that demonstrated an increase in lagging chromosomes and other anaphase abnormalities in mammalian cells after exposure to

TABLE 5   FIDELITY OF MITOSIS OF HUMAN MESOTHELIAL CELLS EXPOSED TO
GLASS FIBERS

Condition	MI[1]	Aberrations[1]				Abnormalities[1]			
		%	D_M	$L_{A/T}$	MP	%	CM	SC	CC
Control	4.9	6.6	3.1	1.2	2.3	3.5	–	0.8	2.7
With glass	6.2	12.9	8.0	1.3	3.7	7.3	2.2	1.7	2.7

[1](MI) Mitotic index; (D_M) chromosome dislocated from mitotic plate; ($L_{A/T}$) lagging chromosomes at anaphase and metaphase; (MP) multipolar metaphase; (CM) chromatin mass; (SC) scattered chromosomes; (CC) chromosome clusters.

asbestos. These types of dysfunction were not observed in human mesothelial cell cultures. In contrast, our results, especially the increase in chromosome clustering, permit us to hypothesize that amosite asbestos fibers disturb the fidelity of mesothelial cell division by inhibiting mitotic tubulin polymerization and/or centriole separation.

The hypothesis that a chromosomal imbalance may be important in tumor development stems from the consistent finding of nonrandom numerical chromosome changes in many forms of cancer (Barrett et al. 1990). When aneuploidy arises in a cell, it may alter cellular regulation by a number of mechanisms. For example, the number of genes and chromosomes will have been altered, and therefore gene dosage effects may cause dysfunction of cellular regulation (Knudson 1985; Oshimura et al. 1988), as was our experimentally observed result with over transcription of PDGF A-chain mRNA. Alternatively, the expression of a recessive gene may be allowed, and this may alter cellular regulation (Knudson 1985; Lee et al. 1987; Vogelstein et al. 1988). Finally, there is the possibility of an indirect effect on the cellular genetic complement, perhaps by an alteration of the rate of DNA synthesis or repair. Both of these processes precede cell division and dysregulation of these functions may therefore induce further genetic instability that in turn could alter cellular regulation (Oshimura et al. 1988). Thus, our preliminary data are consistent with the hypothesis that a major step of fiber-caused neoplastic transformation of human mesothelial cells is the onset of aneuploidy that is caused primarily by disruption of spindle mechanics.

REFERENCES

Assoian, R.K., B.E. Fleurdelys, H.C. Stevenson, P.J. Miller, D.K. Madtes, E.W. Raines, R. Ross, and M.B. Sporn. 1987. Expression and secretion of type beta transforming growth factor by activated human macrophages. *Proc. Natl. Acad. Sci.* **84:** 6020.

Barrett, J.C., T. Tsutsui, T. Tlsty, and M. Oshimura. 1990. Role of genetic instability in carcinogenesis. In *Genetic mechanisms in carcinogenesis and tumor progression* (ed. C.C. Harris and L.A. Liotta), p. 97. Wiley-Liss, New York.

Connell, N.D. and J.G. Rheinwald. 1983. Regulation of the cytoskeleton of mesothelial cells: Reversible loss of keratin and increase of vimentin during rapid growth in culture. *Cell* **34:** 245.

Craighead, J.E. and B.T. Mossman. 1982. The pathogenesis of asbestos-associated diseases. *N. Engl. J. Med.* **306:** 1446.

Gabrielson, E.W., B.I. Gerwin, C.C. Harris, A.B. Roberts, M.B. Sporn, and J.F. Lechner. 1988a. Stimulation of DNA synthesis in cultured primary human mesothelial cells by specific growth factors. *FASEB J.* **2:** 2717.

Gabrielson, E.W., G.M. Rosen, R.C. Grafstrom, K.E. Strauss, M. Miyashita, and C.C. Harris. 1988b. Role of oxygen radicals in 12-0-tetradecanoylphorbol-13-acetate-induced squamous differentiation of cultured normal human bronchial epithelial cells. *Cancer Res.* **48:** 822.

Gerwin, B.I., J.F. Lechner, R.R. Reddel, A.B. Roberts, K.C. Robbins, E.W. Gabrielson, and C.C. Harris. 1987. Comparison of production of transforming growth factor-beta and platelet-derived growth factor by normal human mesothelial cells and mesothelioma cell lines. *Cancer Res.* **47:** 6180.

Gerwin, B.I., C. Betsholtz, K. Linnainmaa, K. Pelin, R.R. Reddel, E.W. Gabrielson, M. Seddon, R. Greenwald, C.C. Harris, and J.F. Lechner. 1990. *In vitro* studies of human mesothelioma. In *Biology, toxicology and carcinogenesis of respiratory epithelium* (ed. D. Thomassen and P. Nettesheim), p. 112. Hemisphere Publishing, New York.

Hartmann, D.P., M.M. Georgian, Y. Oghiso, and E. Kagan. 1984. Enhanced interleukin activity following asbestos inhalation. *Clin. Exp. Immunol.* **55:** 643.

Hesterberg, T.W. and J.C. Barrett. 1985. Induction by asbestos fibers of anaphase abnormalities: Mechanism for aneuploidy induction and possibly carcinogenesis. *Carcinogenesis* **6:** 473.

Ke, Y., R.R. Reddel, B.I. Gerwin, H.K. Reddel, A.N.A. Somers, M.G. McMenamin, M.A. LaVeck, R. Stahel, J.F. Lechner, and C.C. Harris. 1989. Establishment of a human in vitro mesothelial cell model system for investigating mechanisms of asbestos-induced mesothelioma. *Am. J. Pathol.* **134:** 979.

Knudson, A.G., Jr. 1985. Hereditary cancer, oncogenes, and antioncogenes. *Cancer Res.* **45:** 1437.

Kumar, R.K., R.A. Bennett, and A.R. Brody. 1988. A homologue of platelet-derived growth factor produced by rat alveolar macrophages. *FASEB J.* **2:** 2272.

Laemmli, U.K. 1970. Cleavage of structural proteins during the assembly of the head of bacteriophage T4. *Nature* **227:** 680.

LaRocca, P.J. and J.G. Rheinwald. 1985. Anchorage-independent growth of normal human mesothelial cells: A sensitive bioassay for EGF which discloses the absence of this factor in fetal calf serum. *In Vitro* **21:** 67.

LaVeck, M.A., A.N.A. Somers, L.L. Moore, B.I. Gerwin, and J.F. Lechner. 1988. Dissimilar peptide growth factors can induce normal human mesothelial cell multiplication. *In Vitro* **24:** 1077.

Lechner, J.F., M.A. LaVeck, B.I. Gerwin, and E.A. Matis. 1989. Differential responses to growth factors by normal human mesothelial cultures from individual donors. *J. Cell. Physiol.* **139:** 295.

Lechner, J.F., T. Tokiwa, H. Yeager, Jr., and C.C. Harris. 1985a. Asbestos-associated chromosomal changes in human mesothelial cells. *NATO ASI Ser. Ser. G Ecol. Sci.* **3:** 197.

Lechner, J.F., A. Haugen, T. Tokiwa, B.F. Trump, and C.C. Harris. 1983. Effects of asbestos and carcinogenic metals on cultured human bronchial epithelium. In *Human carcinogenesis* (ed. C.C. Harris and H. Autrup), p. 561. Academic Press, New York.

Lechner, J.F., T. Tokiwa, M.A. LaVeck, W.F. Benedict, S.P. Banks-Schlegel, H. Yeager, Jr., A. Banerjee, and C.C. Harris. 1985b. Asbestos-associated chromosomal changes in human mesothelial cells. *Proc. Natl. Acad. Sci.* **82:** 3884.

Lee, W.H., R. Bookstein, F. Hong, L.J. Young, J.Y. Shew, and E.Y Lee. 1987. Human retinoblastoma susceptibility gene: Cloning, identification, and sequence. *Science* **235:** 1394.

Linnainmaa, K., B.I. Gerwin, K. Pelin, K. Jantuene, M.A. LaVeck, J.F. Lechner, and C.C. Harris. 1986. Asbestos-induced mesothelioma and chromosomal abnormalities in human mesothelial cells in vitro. In *The changing nature of work and the work place*, p. 119 National Institute for Occupational Safety and Health, Cincinnati, Ohio.

Mossman, B.T. and J.P. Marsh. 1989. Evidence supporting a role for active oxygen species in asbestos-induced toxicity and lung disease. *Environ. Health Perspect.* **81:** 91.

Nathan, C.F. 1987. Secretory products of macrophages. *J. Clin. Invest.* **79:** 319.

Oshimura, M., M. Koi, N. Ozawa, O. Sugawara, P.W. Lamb, and J.C. Barrett. 1988. Role of chromosome loss in ras/myc-induced Syrian hamster tumors. *Cancer Res.* **48:** 1623.

Parry, E.M. 1985. Tests for effects on mitosis and mitotic spindle in Chinese hamster primary liver cells (CH 1-L) in culture. In *Progress in mutation research 5* (ed. J. Ashbey and F.J. de Serres), p

479. Elsevier, Amsterdam.

Parry, E.M., N. Danford, and J.M. Parry. 1982. Differential staining of chromosomes and spindle and its use as an assay for determining the effect of diethylstilboestrol on cultured mammalian cells. *Mutat. Res.* **105**: 243.

Parry, J.M., N. Danford, and E.M. Parry. 1984. *In vitro* techniques for the detection of chemicals capable of inducing mitotic chromosome aneuploidy. *Altern. Lab. Anim.* **11**: 117.

Sporn, M.B. and G.J. Todaro. 1980. Autocrine secretion and malignant transformation of cells. *N. Engl. J. Med.* **303**: 878.

Van der Meeren, A., B.I. Gerwin, M. Seddon, C. Betsholtz, J.F. Lechner, and C.C. Harris. 1990. The oncogenic potential of overexpression of PDGF-A and -B chain genes in immortalized, nontumorigenic, human mesothelial cells. *Proc. Am. Assoc. Cancer Res.* **31**: 52.

van Zoelen, E.J., T.M. van Oostwaard, and S.W. de Laat. 1986. Transforming growth factor-beta and retinoic acid modulate phenotypic transformation of normal rat kidney cells induced by epidermal growth factor and platelet-derived growth factor. *J. Biol. Chem.* **261**: 5003.

van Zoelen, E.J., T.M. van Oostwaard, P.T. van der Saag, and S.W. de Laat. 1985. Phenotypic transformation of normal rat kidney cells in a growth-factor-defined medium: Induction by a neuroblastoma-derived transforming growth factor independently of the EGF receptor. *J. Cell. Physiol.* **123**: 151.

Vogelstein, B., E.R. Fearon, S.R. Hamilton, S.E. Kern, A.C. Preisinger, N. Leppert, Y. Nakamura, R. White, A.M. Smits, and J.L. Bos. 1988. Genetic alterations during colorectal-tumor development. *N. Engl. J. Med.* **319**: 525.

Wagner, J.C., G. Berry, R.J. Hill, D.E. Munday, and J.W. Skidmore. 1980. Animal experiments with man-made mineral fibres. In *Biological effects of mineral fibres* (ed. J.C. Wagner), p. 361. International Agency for Research on Cancer, Lyon, France.

Wang, N.S., M.C. Jaurand, L. Magne, L. Kheuang, M.C. Pinchon, and J. Bignon. 1987. The interactions between asbestos fibers and metaphase chromosomes of rat pleural mesothelial cells in culture. A scanning and transmission electron microscopic study. *Am. J. Pathol.* **126**: 343.

Wu, Y.J., L.M. Parker, N.E. Binder, M.A. Beckett, J.H. Sinard, C.T. Griffiths, and J.G. Rheinwald. 1982. The mesothelial keratins: A new family of cytoskeletal proteins identified in cultured mesothelial cells and nonkeratinizing epithelia. *Cell* **31**: 693.

Neoplastic Transformation of Rodent Cells

**M.-C. Jaurand, L. Saint-Etienne, A. Van der Meeren,
S. Endo-Capron, A. Renier, and J. Bignon**
*Laboratory of Cellular and Molecular Toxicology, INSERM U 139
94010 Créteil Cedex, France*

INTRODUCTION

Assessment of the neoplastic transformation of rodent cells in vitro is largely used to predict the carcinogenic potency of chemicals (Douglas 1984). This method provides evidence that an agent can be carcinogenic to humans. In addition, cell transformation can be studied in terms of description of the cellular and molecular events involved in cell transformation. Thus, the observation of cell transformation by an agent and the study of the cellular and molecular events involved in cell transformation provide clues on the mechanism by which a carcinogen can generate the important steps in cell transformation.

Several cell systems have been used to assess the neoplastic potency of asbestos fibers and determine their mechanisms of action; they include classical models that have been tested with different carcinogens and new cell systems that have been developed with target cells of asbestos fibers. From the data published in the literature, either morphological or neoplastic transformation of rodent cells by fibers has been assessed using four different cell types, including Syrian hamster embryo (SHE) cells, two types of mice fibroblasts (C3H/10T1/2 and BALB3T3). All three consisted in the classical previously validated cell systems. In addition, a new model of rat pleural mesothelial cells (RPMC) has been developed because of the well-known relationship between asbestos exposure and mesothelioma occurrence in populations exposed to asbestos.

Cellular and Molecular Aspects of Fiber Carcinogenesis
Copyright 1991 Cold Spring Harbor Laboratory Press 0-87969-361-4/91 $1.00 + 00   131

The different models have clearly demonstrated that asbestos fibers are potentially carcinogenic and transform rodent cells, in agreement with the experimental in vivo findings. In these models, cell transformation has been assessed by different endpoints: colony morphology in liquid medium, growth in soft agar, and/or tumorigenicity in athymic nude mice. From data obtained with different cell types, it appears that asbestos may play a role in inducing chromosomal mutations and may act at the first stages of cell transformation. When asbestos has been continuously applied to mesothelial cells in an attempt to mimic the fiber persistency, an enhancement of the probability of cell transformation has been observed. When asbestos has been applied with chemical carcinogens in an attempt to mimic synergy with tobacco smoke, a cocarcinogenic effect has not always been found. These models provide pertinent information on the possible mechanisms of action of asbestos.

ASBESTOS FIBERS MAY TRANSFORM RODENT CELLS

Morphological transformation of rodent cells in the classical systems is detected by different endpoints, either the focus formation on a monolayer or the occurrence of abnormal colonies in a liquid medium after plating at low density. In addition, growth in soft agar and tumorigenesis in nude mice can be used for a better characterization of the stage of transformation. These methods have also been applied to the RPMC system; it has been found that the observation of abnormal colonies at low density, growth in soft agar, and subcutaneous cell inoculation into athymic nude mice were efficient methods to assess cell transformation. Colonies in a liquid medium were classified in four classes according to the importance (surface and number of layers) of the lack of contact inhibition between cells (Paterour et al. 1985).

Table 1 summarizes the results obtained with the different cell types. There is a general agreement to conclude that asbestos transforms rodent cells, but in some experiments, no or only a low transformation was detected in the absence of added cocarcinogen with the C3H/10T1/2 test system and crocidolite.

TABLE 1 *SUMMARY OF TRANSFORMATION ASSAYS WITH RODENT CELLS*

Assay	Transformation[a]		Synergy	
	crocidolite	chrysotile	B(a)P	other
SHE	+	+	+/−	− (UV)
C3H/10T1/2	−/[+][b]	n.t.[c]	+	+ (gamma rays)
BALB3T3	+	+		
RPMC	[+][d]	+	−	

[a]The positivity is taken into consideration only on a qualitative basis. No attempt is made to compare crocidolite with chrysotile.
[b]Not significant, low rate.
[c]n.t. indicates not tested.
[d]Low rate (S. Endo-Capron and M.-C. Jaurand, unpubl.).

C3H/10T1/2 Model: Contribution to the Study of Cocarcinogenesis and Questions on the Role of Oxygen Derivatives

C3H cells were not morphologically transformed by crocidolite at the experimental doses of 5 µg/ml (Brown et al. 1983; Hei et al. 1984, 1985). However, a positive cocarcinogenic effect has been detected with a chemical carcinogen, such as benzo[a]pyrene (B[a]P), and with gamma rays (Brown et al. 1983; Hei et al. 1984, 1985). In parallel studies, Hei et al. (1984) studied the promoting activity of asbestos by irradiating the cells first, followed 3 days later by a continuous treatment with a smaller dose of asbestos fibers (0.1 or 1 µg/ml), and observed a negative promoting effect.

These results are interesting because it has been reported previously that C3H/10T1/2 cells can be transformed by oxygen derivatives that are produced either by the xanthine-xanthine oxidase system (Zimmerman and Cerutti 1984) or by oxygen derivatives produced by 12-O-tetradecanoylphorbol-13-acetate (TPA)-treated neutrophils (Weitzman et al. 1985). Since it has been reported elsewhere that asbestos, especially crocidolite, produces oxygen derivatives (Weitzman and Graceffa 1984; Zalma et al. 1987) and triggers macrophages or tracheal cells to produce such molecules (Goodglick and Kane 1986; Mossman et al. 1986; Hansen and Mossman 1987), the results would suggest that oxiradicals produced by the fibers should be unable to exert their effects. There are at least two possible explanations to account for this observation: First, the amount of radicals produced is insufficient to detect a transformation; and second, formation of radicals, which needs the availability of reduced iron, is impaired by the oxidation of the iron present at the fiber surface, as emphasized by Zalma et al. (1987). Moreover, these experiments suggest that coculture studies involving macrophages or radical producer cells and test cells should be useful in studying the role of asbestos-induced oxygen derivatives.

BALB3T3 Model: Some Clues on the Activity of Asbestos in Multistage Carcinogenesis

The report using the BALB3T3 assay is the only study where a classical promoter, such as TPA, has been tested (Lu et al. 1988). The results indicate that both asbestos fiber types, chrysotile and crocidolite, transform the cells but at different dose levels. On a per weight basis, lower doses of chrysotile are necessary to transform BALB3T3 cells when compared with crocidolite. When tested as initiators with TPA as the promoter, asbestos exhibited initiating activities, and the data suggest that chrysotile is an initiator, whereas crocidolite has only an initiating-like effect. These experiments have concentrated on the initiating activity of asbestos fibers and have not tested the promoting activity. Nevertheless, they indicated that chrysotile may be a complete carcinogen. In view of the numerous data on the clastogenicity and chromosomal effects of asbestos on rodent cells (for review, see Jaurand 1989), these results strongly suggest that the initiating activity may result from the effects of asbestos on the genetic material.

SHE Cell Studies: A Triple Contribution to the Mechanisms of Asbestos Carcinogenesis

First contribution: evidence of transformation. Three studies have reported a morphological transformation of SHE cells following treatment with asbestos (DiPaolo et al. 1983; Hesterberg and Barrett 1984; Mikalsen et al. 1988) as well as neoplastic transformation (Koi and Barrett 1986; Gilmer et al. 1988). In some studies, asbestos was not the only fiber type producing cell transformation; special purpose glass fibers (code 100 and 110) were also efficient. The effect of an association with another chemical carcinogen such as B[a]P was positive in the investigation reported by Di Paolo et al. (1983), whereas no synergy has been detected by Mikalsen et al. (1988). As discussed by these latter investigators, the discrepancies may be reflected in the method used to prepare the fibers.

Second contribution: role of the fiber parameters. The SHE cell model provided a better understanding of the mechanisms of cell transformation by giving information on the role of certain fiber parameters accounting for cell transformation. From animal data, it is known that the carcinogenic effect of asbestos is dependent on the fiber size, with long fibers being more potent than short fibers (Stanton et al. 1977; Davis et al. 1978; Jaurand et al. 1987). In in vitro, this effect has also been observed, since milled chrysotile and milled glass fibers, despite a higher number of fibers on a per weight basis, were less efficient in transforming SHE cells than their unmilled counterparts (Hesterberg and Barrett 1984).

An explanation of this size dependence of the transformation has been given by further investigations carried out with glass fibers (Hesterberg et al. 1986). It has been observed that SHE cells preferentially ingested long fibers, since there was an increase in the mean length of the ingested fibers when compared with the mean length of the fibers in the sample. Moreover, despite a higher number of short fibers ingested in comparison with long fibers, a lower transformation rate has been observed. Thus, a given number of short fibers is less transforming than an equivalent number of long fibers. Despite the fact that these assays have been performed with glass fibers, an extrapolation to asbestos fibers can be made.

The mechanisms sustaining this cell transformation can involve chromosome missegregation. As reported elsewhere with different cell types, including SHE cells, the formation of abnormal anaphases follows the treatment of cells with asbestos (Hesterberg and Barrett 1985; Verschaeve et al. 1985; Palekar et al. 1987); it may result in the formation of aneuploid and polyploid cells as reported previously for many cell types (for review, see Jaurand 1989). Chromosome missegregation is an important event in SHE cell transformation, as reported previously in studies on the neoplastic progression of SHE cells in vitro; aneuploidy has been detected in asbestos-treated SHE cells (Oshimura et al. 1984). It is conceivable that the longer the fibers, the higher the probability that they interact with microtubules or with chromosomes.

Long versus short fibers have also differential effects in their ability to induce macrophages to produce radicals (Hansen and Mossman 1987). Whether this mechanism is an additional way for other asbestos-treated cells to respond to asbestos remains unknown.

Third contribution: molecular events associated with SHE cell transformation. It has been demonstrated that neoplastic transformation of SHE cells is a progressive process where normal cells reach a neoplastic state through a preneoplastic state (Barrett 1980; Crawford et al. 1983). This later state is characterized by an immortalization and is associated with phenotypical changes, but the cells are not tumorigenic nor do they grow in soft agar. The neoplastic progression is associated with chromosomal and genetic changes. Preneoplastic cells are aneuploid, and some clones obtained shortly after treatment with asbestos exhibit an aneuploidy characterized by a trisomy of chromosome 11 (Oshimura et al. 1986). Somatic hybridization methods have shown that transformed cells may have lost a tumor-suppressor gene (see Barrett, this volume). Some transformed cells have an activated *ras*, but other oncogenes may be involved in cell transformation (Gilmer et al. 1988).

The involvement of oncogenes in SHE cell transformation has been confirmed by transfection experiments; transfection of normal cells with a plasmid containing v-*myc* or v-Ha-*ras* does not produce tumorigenic cells, but the association of both genes results in a tumorigenic potency in athymic nude mice (Thomassen et al. 1985). When preneoplastic cells, including asbestos-treated cells are transfected with v-Ha-*ras*, tumorigenic cells are obtained (Koi and Barrett 1986). These observations indicate that asbestos fibers can exert an effect at early stages rendering the cells sensitive to the action of critical genes. Moreover, analyses of the *ras* oncogene in asbestos-treated cells have shown that some cell lines contained an activated form of the gene (Gilmer et al. 1988). In other studies, it has been observed that some cell lines derived from asbestos-treated cells have lost a suppressor gene (Koi and Barrett 1986). These observations do not imply that asbestos has induced mutations, although it may suggest this conclusion, but it indicates that asbestos fibers have at least committed cells to progress through transformation.

RPMC: A New Model in Fair Agreement with the Classical Models

The transformation of RPMC has been assessed using the short-term transformation assay designed with the other cell types. Moreover, a long-term assay has been designed in an attempt to mimic the persistence of the fibers in the biological milieu.

Treatment of RPMC with 1 µg/cm^2 of Rhodesian chrysotile asbestos resulted in the formation of abnormal colonies in a liquid medium. The colonies were classified according to the level of loss of contact inhibition between cells, as mentioned above. A significant enhancement of the transformation frequency has been detected in the treated cultures, which is in agreement with other studies described above. However, no significant synergy between chrysotile and B[a]P has been detected (Jaurand et al. 1988). The lack of synergy is difficult to interpret in comparison with the other studies because the fiber sample was different (other studies have concerned Canadian chrysotile or amphiboles), and each agent at the concentration used was able to produce a significant rate of transformants. These results could be considered as being in agreement with the lack of synergy observed in humans between asbestos exposure and tobacco consumption. However, several remarks can be made: First, chemicals from tobacco smoke can be metabolized by lung cells before reaching the pleura and can exert their effects in other cells, as suggested by the prevalence of lung cancer in smokers; second, B[a]P is not the unique component of tobacco smoke, and use of other substances could be more relevant.

Neoplastic transformation of RPMC has been assessed

using a long-term model, where the fibers were applied repetitively to the cell cultures to mimic the effect of the fiber persistence within the tissue. Actually, despite the clearance mechanisms, the fibers remain for a certain time in the lung tissue and could therefore exert their effect for a certain period of time.

In a first set of experiments, the study has been designed to determine the promoting capacity of asbestos (Paterour et al. 1985). B[a]P has been used as the initiator, since previous studies had demonstrated its transforming potency. According to the protocol, RPMC received a unique application of B[a]P followed by a repetitive (approximately weekly) treatment with chrysotile fibers. Under these conditions, abnormal colonies in liquid medium were detected by the method of plating at low density. Colonies exhibiting piled up cells appeared after about 32 passages both in B[a]P-treated cultures and in chrysotile-treated cultures, but the addition of chrysotile to the B[a]P-treated cells did not enhance the transformation frequency. The results suggested that chrysotile asbestos acted, under these conditions, as a complete carcinogen.

RPMC and the Long-term Model

Another experiment has been performed to confirm the transforming potency of asbestos and to study the stages of cell transformation under the specific conditions described previously (Saint-Etienne et al. 1989). In this experiment, B[a]P has been omitted, but a new series of cells receiving only one treatment has been made. Therefore, three series were cultured: repetitively treated, treated once, and untreated cultures. In these series of experiments, neoplastic transformation has been characterized by the detection of the anchorage independence and of tumorigenesis following subcutaneous inoculation into nude mice. Several results have been found: (1) RPMC, having received repetitive treatment with chrysotile, exhibited signs of neoplastic transformation sooner than RPMC having received only one treatment; and (2) untreated RPMC at very late passages exhibited some signs of neoplastic transformation. The results allowed us to suggest some hypotheses to account for the observed effects.

In the untreated, long-term cultures, is there an effect of the number of population doublings? Untreated cultures formed tumors in nude mice when inoculated at passage 75, i.e., a duration of culture of about 1.5 years. After inoculation of 2 x 10^6 cells into nude mice, only 20% of mice formed tumors, and the delay of appearance of the first tumor was 21 weeks. A relationship between delay of tumor formation and number of tumor cells inoculated has been reported previously with other cell systems (Freedman and Shin 1978). Figure 1 shows that similar relationship may be obtained by the inoculation of neoplastic RPMC. Two hypotheses can therefore be made to account for the delay between time of cell inoculation into nude mice and tumor appearance; first, this phenomenon is related to the number of fully neoplastic cells, and second, it is due to the fact that the inoculated cells are only preneoplastic

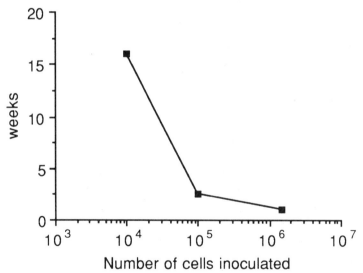

FIGURE 1 Relationship between delay to obtain 50% of tumors according to the number of cells subcutaneously inoculated into nude mice. The inoculated RPMC were derived from an agar colony further expanded in the absence of asbestos, according to standard culturing in liquid medium. This colony was obtained from a 60-passages-old culture of RPMC with chrysotile repetitively treated. Inoculation of 10^6 cells resulted in the formation of stable tumors in 100% of the nude mice.

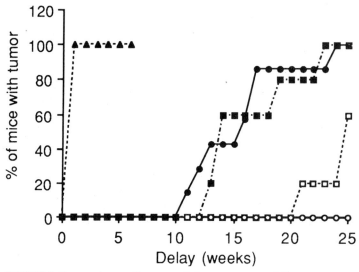

FIGURE 2 Percentage of mice exhibiting tumor following inoculation of 1.5 x 10⁶ RPMC according to the delay after inoculation. Untreated cells: (open boxes) passage 75; (open circles) passage 51. Cells having received repetitive chrysotile treatment: (closed triangles) passage 75; (closed circles) passage 53; (closed boxes) passage 46.

and have to mature. When the first hypothesis is taken into consideration, it can be deduced from Figure 1 that approximately 0.2% of the inoculated cells were neoplastic, whereas no tumorigenicity was observed at passage 51 (Fig. 2).

The so-called spontaneous transformation might arise from the aging of the culture. Repetitive subculturing for 75 passages makes the cell divide for a high number of rounds. It is known that aging results in an increase of spontaneous tumor occurrences (Ames 1990). The period of time required for neoplastic transformation will depend on the accumulation of a number of events involved in the transformation process, either by simple accumulation of mutation damages or by an accelerated mutation rate. DNA damage is involved in the cell progression toward a neoplastic state. Therefore, the appearance of neoplastic cells in an untreated culture can result from the in vitro aging, as a result of hits derived from the continuous subculturing or from other reasons.

The effect of asbestos on long-term cultures. The repetitive application of chrysotile on RPMC cultures resulted in the formation of abnormal colonies and anchorage-independence as early as passage 40. Moreover, tumorigenesis has been observed at passage 46 (not tested before). After a delay of 13 weeks following inoculation, 50% of the inoculated mice exhibited tumors. If the same assumptions concerning the relationship between tumor formation and number of cells inoculated was made, a rate of 5% of tumor cells can be present in the inoculated culture. This strongly contrasts with the untreated cells where no tumor was induced at passage 51. Moreover, at the same "age" as the untreated cells (passage 75), all the cells were neoplastic, since 100% of tumors were observed within 1 week (Fig. 2).

Cultures having received only one chrysotile treatment showed intermediate features. In effect, if 100% of the inoculated mice formed tumors following inoculation at passage 75, no tumors were detected at passage 46 in these series, in contrast with the repetitively treated cultures. These results allow us to establish an order of cell transformation: repetitively treated cultures > cultures treated once >> untreated cultures. It is therefore suggested that asbestos enhances the rate of transformation and has an aging-like effect. Asbestos may accelerate the process of cell transformation; this may be related to the mutagenic effect, in a large sense, of the fibers. Experiments are now in progress to characterize the oncogenes activated in the different series. The involvement of epidermal-growth-factor-like growth factors has been suggested previously (Van der Meeren et al. 1988).

A suggested mechanism for asbestos-induced RPMC transformation. From the data that was reported, the following mechanism can be suggested. Asbestos interacts with microtubules and chromosomes (Wang et al. 1987). These events may play a role in the induction of cell aneuploidy. It has been found that, 48 hours after treatment with 1 $\mu g/cm^2$ of Canadian chrysotile fibers, RPMC exhibited a significant trisomy of chromosome 1 (22% vs. 6% in control cells). In the long-term experiment described above, after one treatment with Rhode-

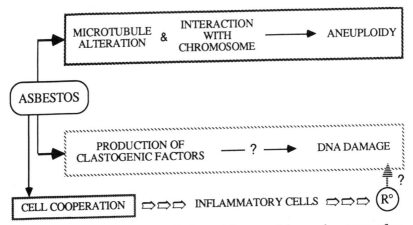

FIGURE 3 Schematic representation of the possible mechanisms of action of asbestos on RPMC.

sian chrysotile and ten additional passages without fibers, 68% of the metaphases exhibited the trisomy against 30% in the untreated cells. Similar observations with mesothelial cells in asbestos-treated cells have been reported previously by other investigators (Palekar et al. 1989) or in spontaneous mesothelioma (Walker et al. 1991). By analogy with what has been suggested previously (Barrett et al. 1987), Figure 3 summarizes the present hypotheses. In addition to chromosome mutations, asbestos may commit cells to produce DNA-damaging factors, and the fibers themselves are able to produce radicals as mentioned above. Human mesothelial cells did not produce OH· following treatment with amosite (Gabrielson et al. 1986), but the cells might release clastogenic factors, as was demonstrated with rat cells (M.-C. Jaurand, unpubl.). These molecules may produce DNA damage, but until now a direct involvement of these molecules in the damage of the mesothelial cell genome has not been reported.

There is an additional mechanism that could take a part in the carcinogenesis of asbestos: A cell cooperation can be suggested. Recently, it has been reported that treated mesothelial cells release chemotactic factors for polymorphonuclear neutrophils (PMN) (Antony et al. 1989). PMN might in turn release

DNA-damaging molecules, such as radicals. Using the method of intrapleural inoculation of fibers, which is one usually performed to assess the carcinogenic potency of fibers, an influx of macrophages and inflammatory cells are observed in the pleural space shortly after inoculation. Although no proof has been brought of the role of this process, it seems that the involvement of a cell cooperation may be also considered.

The mechanisms whereby asbestos transforms cells are still unclear, and efforts have to be made to understand better their mechanism of action. It is clear that morphological and neoplastic transformation of rodent cells by asbestos has been observed with several cell types, including the target mesothelial cells. However, at the concentrations used, C3H/10T1/2 cells were not significantly morphologically transformed in the absence of another carcinogen. Both fiber types were efficient but at different doses, and it is not the aim of this paper to compare their transforming potency. SHE cells, BALB3T3 cells, and RPMC have normal chromosome numbers in contrast with C3H/10T1/2 cells, which have an abnormal karyotype (Brouty-Boye et al. 1982). If aneuploidy is a critical event in asbestos-induced neoplastic transformation, it is possible that this characteristic impairs the occurrence of such an event. The observation of a neoplastic transformation in independent cell types and independent studies reinforces the conclusion of the transforming potency of asbestos. In the mesothelial cell model, even one treatment with chrysotile is sufficient to accelerate cell transformation strongly but is much less efficient than a continuous exposure. It can be assumed that a single exposure should be sufficient to produce a cell transformation but that additional events should have to occur. However, it must also be emphasized that the probability of cell transformation should be distinguished from the probability of tumor formation, which is dependent on other parameters playing a role at the organ or at the body level (e.g., clearance of the fibers and immunological survey).

ACKNOWLEDGMENT

The authors thank Mrs. Catherine Vaslin for typing the manuscript.

REFERENCES

Ames, B.N. 1990. Mutagenesis and carcinogenesis: Endogenous and exogenous factors. *Environ. Mol. Mutagen.* **16:** 66.

Antony, V.B., C.L. Owen, and K.J. Hadley. 1989. Pleural mesothelial cells stimulated by asbestos release chemotactic activity for neutrophils in vitro. *Am. Rev. Respir. Dis.* **139:** 199.

Barrett, J.C. 1980. A preneoplastic stage in the spontaneous neoplastic transformation of Syrian hamster embryo cells in culture. *Cancer Res.* **40:** 91.

Barrett, J.C., O. Mitsuo, N. Tanaka, and T. Tsutsui. 1987. Genetic and epigenetic mechanisms of presumed nongenotoxic carcinogens. *Banbury Rep.* **25:** 311.

Brouty-Boye, D., I. Gresser, and M.T. Bandu. 1982. Stability of the phenotypic reversion of X-ray transformed C3H/10T1/2 cells depends on cellular proliferation after subcultivation at low cell density. *Carcinogenesis* **3:** 1057.

Brown, R.C., A. Poole, and G.T.A. Fleming. 1983. The influence of asbestos dust on the oncogenic transformation of C3H 10 T1/2 cells. *Cancer Lett.* **18:** 221.

Crawford, B.D., J.C. Barrett, and P.O.P. Ts'o. 1983. Neoplastic conversion of preneoplastic Syrian hamster cells: Rate estimation by fluctuation analysis. *Mol. Cell. Biol.* **3:** 931.

Davis, J.M.G., S.T. Beckett, R.E. Bolton, P. Collings, and A.P. Middleton. 1978. Mass and number of fibers in the pathogenesis of asbestos-related lung disease in rats. *Br. J. Cancer* **37:** 673.

Di Paolo, J.A., A.J. De Marinis, and J. Doniger. 1983. Asbestos and benzo(a)pyrene synergism in the transformation of Syrian hamster embryo cells. *Pharmacology* **27:** 65.

Douglas, J.F., ed. 1984. *Carcinogenesis and mutagenesis testing.* Humana Press, Clifton, New Jersey.

Freedman, V.H. and S. Shin. 1978. use of nude mice for studies on the tumorigenicity of animal cells. In *The nude mouse in experimental and clinical research* (ed. J. Fogh and B.C. Giovanella), p. 353. Academic Press, New York.

Gabrielson, E.W., G.M. Rosen, R.C. Grafstrom, K.E. Strauss, and C.C. Harris. 1986. Studies on the role of oxygen radicals in asbestos-induced cytopathology of cultured human lung mesothelial cells. *Carcinogenesis* **7:** 1161.

Gilmer, T.M., L.A. Annab, and J.C. Barrett. 1988. Characterization of activated protooncogenes in chemically transformed Syrian hamster embryo-cells. *Mol. Carcinog.* **1:** 180.

Goodglick, L.A. and A.B. Kane. 1986. Role of reactive oxygen metabolites in crocidolite asbestos toxicity to mouse macrophages. *Cancer Res.* **46:** 5558.

Hansen, K. and B.T. Mossman. 1987. Generation of superoxide (O_2^{-}) from aveolar macrophages exposed to asbestiform and non fibrous particles. *Cancer Res.* **47:** 1681.

Hei, T.K., E.J. Hall, and R.S. Osmak. 1984. Asbestos, radiation and oncogenic transformation. *Br. J. Cancer* **50:** 717.

Hei, T.K., C.R. Geard, R.S. Osmak, and M. Travisano. 1985. Correlation of in vitro genotoxicity and oncogenicity induced by radiation and asbestos fibers. *Br. J. Cancer* **52:** 591.

Hesterberg, T.W. and J.C. Barrett. 1984. Dependence of asbestos and mineral dust-induced transformation of mammalian cells in culture on fiber dimension. *Cancer Res.* **44:** 2170.

————. 1985. Induction by asbestos fibers of anaphase abnormalities: Mechanism for aneuploidy induction and possibly carcinogenesis. *Carcinogenesis* **6:** 473.

Hesterberg, T.W., C.J. Butterick, M. Oshimura, A.R. Brody, and J.C. Barrett. 1986. Role of phagocytosis in Syrian hamster cell transformation and cytogenetic effects induced by asbestos and short and long glass fibers. *Cancer Res.* **46:** 5795.

Jaurand, M.C. 1989. A particulate state carcinogenesis: Recent data on the mechanism of action of fibres. *IARC Sci. Publ.* **90:** 54.

Jaurand, M.C., J. Fleury, G. Monchaux, M. Nebut, and J. Bignon. 1987. Pleural carcinogenic potency (asbestos, attapulgite) and their cytotoxicity on cultured cells. *J. Natl. Cancer Inst.* **79:** 797.

Jaurand, M.C., A. Renier, A. Gaudichet, L. Kheuang, L. Magne, and J. Bignon. 1988. Short-term tests for the evaluation of potential cancer risk of modified asbestos fibers. *Ann. N.Y. Acad. Sci.* **534:** 741.

Koi, M. and J.C. Barrett. 1986. Loss of tumor-suppressive function during chemically induced neoplastic progression of Syrian hamster embryo cells. *Proc. Natl. Acad. Sci.* **8:** 5992.

Lu, Y.P., C. Lasne, R. Lowy, and I. Chouroulinkov. 1988. Use of orthogonal design methods to study the synergistic effects of asbestos fibres and 12-0-tetradecanoylphorbol-13-acetate (TPA) in the BALB/3T3 cell transformation. *Mutagenesis* **3:** 355.

Mikalsen, S.O., E. Rivedal, and T. Sanner. 1988. Morphological transformation of Syrian hamster embryo cells induced by mineral fibers and the allegated enhancement of benzo(a)pyrene. *Carcinogenesis* **9:** 891.

Mossman, B.T., J.P. Marsh, and M.A. Shatos. 1986. Alteration of superoxide dimutase activity in tracheal epithelial cells by asbestos and inhibition of cytotoxicity by antioxidants. *Lab. Invest.* **54:** 204.

Oshimura, W., T.W. Hesterberg, and J.C. Barrett. 1986. An early, non random karyotypic change in immortal Syrian hamster cell lines transformed by asbestos: Trisomy of chromosome 11. *Cancer Genet. Cytogenet.* **22:** 225.

Oshimura, W., T.W. Hesterberg, T. Tsutsui, and J.C. Barrett. 1984. Correlation of asbestos-induced cytogenetic effects with cell transformation of Syrian hamster embryo cells in culture. *Cancer Res.* **44:** 5017.

Palekar, L.D., J.F. Eyre, and D.L. Coffin. 1989. Chromosomal changes associated with tumorigenic mineral fibres. In *Biological interaction of inhaled mineral fibers and cigarette smoke* (ed. A.P. Wehner), p. 355. Battelle Press, Columbus, Ohio.

Palekar, L.D., J.F. Eyre, B.M. Most, and D.L. Coffin. 1987. Metaphase and anaphase analysis of V79 cells exposed to erionite, UICC chrysotile and UICC crocidolite. *Carcinogenesis* **8:** 553.

Paterour, M.J., J. Bignon, and M.C. Jaurand. 1985. In vitro transformation of rat pleural mesothelial cells by chrysotile fibres and/or benzo(a)pyrene. *Carcinogenesis* **6:** 523.

Saint-Etienne, L., M. Nebut, J. Fleury-Feith, M.J. Paterour, L. Kheuang, J. Bignon, and M.C. Jaurand. 1989. Occurrence and morphology of tumours induced in nude mice transplanted with pleural mesothelial cells in vitro treated with chrysotile or benzo3-4 pyrene. In *Effects of mineral dusts* (ed. B.T. Mossman and R.O. Begin), vol. H30, p. 415. Springer-Verlag, Berlin.

Stanton, M.F., M. Layard, A. Tegeris, E. Miller, M. May, and E. Kent. 1977. Carcinogenicity of fibrous glass: Pleural response in the rat in relation to fiber dimension. *J. Natl. Cancer Inst.* **58:** 587.

Thomassen, D.G., T.M. Gilmer, L. Annab, and J.C. Barrett. 1985. Evidence for multiple steps in neoplastic transformation of normal and preneoplastic Syrian hamster embryo cells following transfection with Harvey murine sarcoma virus oncogene (v-Ha-*ras*). *Cancer Res.* **45:** 726.

Van der Meeren, A., F. Levy, J. Bignon, and M.C. Jaurand. 1988. Growth of normal and neoplastic rat pleural mesothelial cells in the presence of conditioned medium from neoplastic mesothelial cells. *Biol. Cell* **62:** 293.

Verschaeve, L., P. Palmer, and P. In't Veld. 1985. On the uptake and genotoxicity of UICC Rhodesian chrysotile A in human primary lung fibroblasts. *Naturwissenschaften.* **72:** 326.

Walker, C., J. Everitt, E. Bermudez, and K. Funaki. 1991. Involvement of chromosome 1 in rat mesothelial cell transformation. *Toxicologist* (in press).

Wang, N.S., M.C. Jaurand, L. Magne, L. Kheuang, M.C. Pinchon, and J. Bignon. 1987. The interactions between asbestos fibers and metaphase chromosomes of rat pleural mesothelial cells in culture. *Am. J. Pathol.* **126:** 343.

Weitzman, S.A. and P. Graceffa. 1984. Asbestos catalyzes hydroxyl and superoxide radical generation from hydrogen peroxide. *Arch. Biochem. Biophys.* **228:** 373.

Weitzman, S.A., A.B. Weitberg, E.P. Clark, and T.P. Stossel. 1985. Phagocytes as carcinogens: Malignant transformation produced by human neutrophils. *Science* **227:** 1231.

Zalma, R., L. Bonneau, M.C. Jaurand, J. Guignard, and H. Pezerat. 1987. Formation of oxy-radicals by oxygen reduction arising from the surface activity of asbestos. *Can. J. Chem.* **65:** 2338.

Zimmerman, R. and P. Cerutti. 1984. Active oxygen acts as a promoter of transformation in mouse embryo C3H/10T1/2/C18 fibroblasts. *Proc. Natl. Acad. Sci.* **81:** 2085.

Growth Factor and Receptor Expression by Mesothelial Cells: A Comparison between Rodents and Humans

C. Walker, E. Bermudez, and J. Everitt
Chemical Industry Institute of Toxicology
Research Triangle Park, North Carolina 27709

INTRODUCTION

The pathogenesis of mesothelioma induced by mineral fibers, such as asbestos, is at present ill-defined. Although it is clear that several types of cells may be targets for asbestos-induced injury (Jaurand 1989), the mechanism by which this injury is translated into a transforming event at the level of the mesothelial cell remains to be elucidated. Among recent advances in our understanding of this disease process in man is the knowledge that alterations occur in the expression of growth factors in transformed mesothelial cells (Gerwin et al. 1987; Versnel et al. 1988). Alterations in growth factor response and/or production are frequently observed in many types of transformed cells (Roberts and Sporn 1986) and can result in autocrine stimulation of growth (Sporn and Roberts 1985; Browder et al. 1989). Understanding the function of both endogenous and exogenous growth factors in the biology of normal mesothelial cells will be critical for determining the role that altered growth factor production might play in the neoplastic process.

Of additional concern is the question of how closely the biology of mesothelioma development in other species resembles that in humans. The danger to human health of mineral fibers, such as asbestos, has been clearly recognized for some time. This has led to a search for replacement fibers to be used as asbestos substitutes. The safety of such fibers must be assessed in species other than humans, and rodents such as

Cellular and Molecular Aspects of Fiber Carcinogenesis
Copyright 1991 Cold Spring Harbor Laboratory Press 0-87969-361-4/91 $1.00 + 00

rats and hamsters are frequently used for this purpose. The use of such animals as "human surrogates" must be based on an understanding of the similarity (or dissimilarity) in the development of the rodent endpoints (such as tumor incidence) to man. It is therefore important to compare the biology of rodent and human mesothelial cells and to determine whether the mechanism by which these cells are transformed by mineral fibers is the same or different in the two species. As a first step in this process, we have analyzed the expression of a panel of growth factors and their receptors in normal rat mesothelial cells. This paper summarizes our work and that of other investigators on the characterization of growth factor production and responsiveness in normal rat and human mesothelial cells.

Establishment of Normal Rat Mesothelial Cell Cultures

Jaurand et al. (1981) were the first to develop techniques for the establishment and maintenance of normal rat mesothelial cells in culture. We have modified this technique to isolate cells from the intracostal region of the parietal pleura rather than from the diaphragm, as reported by Jaurand. In our hands, isolation of cells from the intracostal region with high-specific-activity collagenase yields a cell population that is significantly enriched for mesothelial cells with good viability and reduces problems with contamination of myoblast-like cells that occasionally occur in preparations of cells from the diaphragm.

To date, nine independent cultures of rat mesothelial cells have been established. Two of these, M12C1 and M12C2, have been extensively characterized by both light and electron microscopy (Bermudez et al. 1990). Both strains appear normal morphologically and are nontumorigenic when injected into nude mice at late passage (M12C1 passage 33 and M12C2 passage 81). These cell strains have served as the basis for our studies into the biology of normal rat mesothelial cells.

Growth Factor Receptor Expression

Poly(A)$^+$ RNA was isolated from the two normal rat mesothelial cell strains, M12C1 and M12C2. At the level of Northern blot analysis, transcripts for the β-subunit of the platelet-derived growth factor (PDGF) receptor (Fig. 1) were expressed by normal cells. The presence of receptors for PDGF was confirmed with binding studies using ^{125}I-labeled recombinant

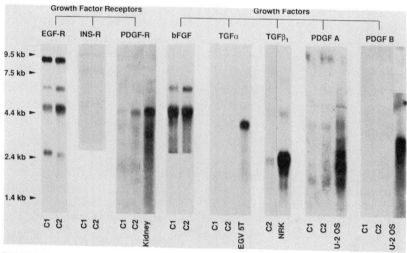

FIGURE 1 Northern blot analysis of poly(A)$^+$ RNA (5 μg/lane) isolated from rat mesothelial cells (M12C1 and M12C2) and controls (rat kidney and the cell lines EGV5T, NRK 52E, and U-2 OS). RNA blotted onto nitrocellulose was probed with radiolabeled DNA probes. Transcript sizes in kilobases for the markers in an RNA ladder standard are indicated by arrowheads. Occasionally, a very diffuse background staining was observed in lanes *C1* and *C2* hybridized to the PDGF A-chain probe. Because of the absence of discrete bands for specific transcripts, the C1 and C2 cells were scored as negative in this assay for PDGF-1 A expression. The following probes were used: insulin receptor pHIR/P12-1 from ATCC, human actin pHF (Gunning et al. 1983) from K. Nelson, rat bFGF RObFGF503 (Shimasaki et al. 1988) from S. Shimasaki, rat TGF-α prTGF$_{0.2}$ (Lee et al. 1985) from D. Lee, murine TGF-β$_1$ sp65Murbas (Derynck et al. 1986) from R. Derynck, human PDGF-A PDGFaD-1 (Betsholtz et al. 1986) from C. Betsholtz, human PDGF-B PSM-1 (Clarke et al. 1984) from M.F. Clarke, a subclone (pGR102) of the murine type B PDGF-R (Yarden et al. 1986) from L.T. Williams, and rat EGF receptor pJH 10.1 (Earp et al. 1988) from H.S. Earp. (Reprinted, with permission, from Bermudez et al. 1990.)

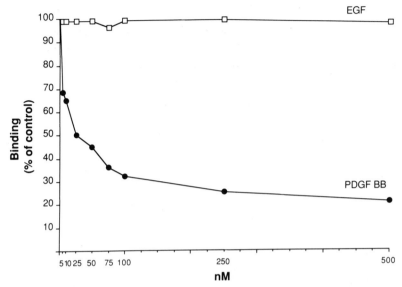

FIGURE 2 Specificity of ^{125}I-labeled PDGF binding to normal rat mesothelial cells. Confluent cell cultures of M12C2 cell strain were incubated 3 hr at 4°C with 0.5 nM ^{125}I-labeled PDGF-BB (Amersham) and various amounts of unlabeled PDGF-BB (Upstate Biotechnology Inc.) or EGF (Collaborative Research). Binding was terminated, and cell bound radioactivity was determined.

PDGF-BB. Binding of PDGF-BB could be competed with cold PDGF-BB (Fig. 2), but not epidermal growth factor (EGF) or heparin, and was saturable (data not shown).

The receptor for EGF was also expressed at the RNA level (Fig. 1). A recent report (Van der Meeren et al. 1990) indicates that normal rat mesothelial cells bind EGF with low affinity and that the growth of these cells can be modulated by exogenous EGF. In addition, insulin receptors were also expressed by both strains of mesothelial cells (Fig. 1).

Expression of Growth Factors

The expression of several growth factors was also examined by Northern blot analysis of mRNA isolated from the rat mesothelial cell strains. No specific transcripts for the ligands for either the PDGF or EGF receptor (PDGF or transforming growth factor [TGF-α], respectively) could be detected. At the level of RNA analysis, it would therefore appear that neither of these growth factors participate in an autocrine loop in normal rat mesothelial cells. The normal cells did express transcripts for TGF-β_1 in very low abundance relative to the rat cell line NRK 52E, which expresses a high level of these transcripts (Fig. 1). In addition, the rat mesothelial cells also expressed transcripts for fibroblast growth factor (FGF) (Fig. 1).

Comparison of the Role of Growth Factors in the Biology of Rat and Human Mesothelial Cells

The expression of growth factors by normal human meso-thelial cells and their responsiveness to various growth factors has been extensively investigated (Table 1). Of particular interest are results on the expression of PDGF. Normal human mesothelial cells express only very low or undetectable amounts of RNA transcripts for the A- and B-chains of this growth factor (Gerwin et al. 1987). Human mesothelial cells are responsive to PDGF-induced stimulation of DNA synthesis, indicating the presence of biologically active receptors on the surface of these cells (Laveck et al. 1988). Interestingly, transformed human mesothelioma cells express abundant RNA transcripts for both the A- and B-chains of PDGF and secrete a PDGF-like mitogenic protein into the media that can be inhibited with a PDGF-specific antibody (Gerwin et al. 1987). These data suggest that PDGF may act as an autocrine growth factor for human mesothelioma cells.

In contrast, in a preliminary report, Jaurand and co-workers describe normal rat mesothelial cells as unresponsive to PDGF (Van der Meeren et al. 1989). However, these cells do bind PDGF-BB homodimers (Fig. 2) and express transcripts for the β-subunit of the PDGF receptor (Fig. 1). No specific transcripts for either the A- or B-chains of PDGF could be detected by Northern blot analysis in normal rat mesothelial cells (Fig. 1). Interestingly, Jaurand and co-workers report that transformed rat mesothelioma cells also do not respond to PDGF (Van der Meeren et al. 1989). If this preliminary observation is

TABLE 1 CHARACTERIZATION OF NORMAL MESOTHELIAL CELLS

	Growth factor expression	Growth factor responsiveness
Human PDGF:	no PDGF-like activity in media conditioned by mesothelial cells (Gerwin et al. 1987)	PDGF-AB/BB: mitogenic (Laveck et al. 1988) TGF-β_1/β_2: mitogenic (Laveck et al. 1988) EGF: mitogenic (Laveck et al. 1988); required for growth (Connell et al. 1983; LaRocca and Rheinwald 1985; Gabrielson et al. 1987)
PDGF-A:	RNA transcripts absent or barely detectable (Gerwin et al. 1987; Versnel et al. 1988)	FGF: mitogenic (Laveck et al. 1988)
PDGF-B:	no detectable expression (Gerwin et al. 1987; Versnel et al. 1988)	IL-1$_\alpha$, IL-1$_\beta$, INF-β, INF-γ, TGF-α (Laveck et al. 1988)
TGF-β:	expression of RNA transcripts and protein (Gerwin et al. 1987	
bFGF:	expression of RNA transcripts (Gerwin et al. 1990)	
mCSF:	expression of RNA transcripts (Demetri et al. 1989)	
G/GMCSF:	inducible by EGF and lymphokines (Demetri et al. 1989)	
Rat PDGF:	no specific transcripts for A or B detected (Bermudez et al. 1990)	PDGF: PDGF-receptor transcripts expressed (Bermudez et al. 1990); specific binding of BB homodimer (C. Walker, unpubl.); no effect on DNA synthesis (Van der Meeren et al. 1989)
TGF-β:	expression of RNA transcripts (Bermudez et al. 1990)	
bFGF:	expression of RNA transcripts (Bermudez et al. 1990)	EGF: inhibits growth (Van der Meeren et al. 1990)
TGF-α:	no transcripts detectable (Bermudez et al. 1990)	

substantiated, it would indicate that a fundamental difference exists in the potential role for PDGF in mesothelioma development in rats and man. If PDGF production by human mesothelioma cells is causally related to transformation of these cells by asbestos, the absence of a role for this growth factor in mesothelioma development in the rat will have implications for the use of this animal model for testing the safety of asbestos substitutes.

In addition to PDGF, rat mesothelial cells also differ from human mesothelial cells in their response to EGF (Table 1). EGF is mitogenic for human mesothelial cells (Laveck et al. 1988), and this growth factor is required for propagation of this cell type in culture (Connell and Rheinwald 1983; LaRocca and Rheinwald 1985; Gabrielson et al. 1987). In contrast, EGF acts to inhibit the growth of normal rat mesothelial cells (Van der Meeren et al. 1990). In a preliminary report, a stimulatory effect of EGF on transformed mesothelioma cells has been reported (Van der Meeren et al. 1989), suggesting that altered EGF responsiveness may be associated with transformation of rat mesothelial cells. EGF receptor transcripts are expressed by normal rat mesothelial cells (Bermudez et al. 1990), but the binding of EGF to this cell type appears to be of low affinity (K_d–1.7 nM) (Van der Meeren et al. 1990). Expression of these low-affinity receptors may be related to the lack of mitogenic response to this growth factor by normal rat mesothelial cells, and a change in the affinity of the EGF receptor for its ligand could play a role in the altered responsiveness of transformed rat mesothelial cells to EGF. TGF-α, which binds to the EGF receptor, is not detectably expressed by normal rat mesothelial cells, but transcripts for TGF-α are expressed by rat mesothelioma cell lines (E. Bermudez, unpubl.), indicating that this growth factor may play a role in the pathogenesis of this disease. Both human and rat mesothelial cells expressed transcripts for FGF and TGF-β_1 (Table 1). Although FGF is mitogenic for human mesothelial cells (Laveck et al. 1988), the response of rat mesothelial cells to this growth factor remains to be determined. Human mesothelial cells also express transcripts for several colony-stimulating factors, but it is not known at this time whether any of these growth factors are expressed by rat mesothelial cells.

DISCUSSION

Significant differences exist between human and rat mesothelial cells, both in the production and the responsiveness to growth factors. PDGF and EGF have very different effects on the growth of human and rat mesothelial cells. In addition, whereas transformed human mesothelial cells express abundant PDGF A- and B-chain transcripts (Gerwin et al. 1987), the expression of these transcripts in either spontaneously transformed or asbestos-transformed rat mesothelial cells has not been observed (C. Walker, unpubl.). The interpretation of this data, with regard to a common mechanism for transformation of rat and human mesothelial cells, awaits information on whether PDGF production by human mesothelial cells is causally related to the disease. Production of other growth factors, such as TGF-α (E. Bermudez, unpubl.) or FGF-like proteins (O'Connell and Rheinwald, this volume) may be involved in transformation of mesothelial cells and may play a similar role in both cell types. An understanding of the commonality of mechanism(s) for transformation of rat and human mesothelial cells will be required in the future for interpreting rodent bioassay data generated in the search for safer fibers for use as asbestos substitutes.

REFERENCES

Bermudez, E., J. Everitt, and C. Walker. 1990. Expression of growth factor and growth factor receptor RNA in rat pleural mesothelial cells in culture. *Exp. Cell Res.* **190:** 91.

Betsholtz, C., A. Johnsson, C. Heldin, B. Westermark, P. Lind, M.S. Urdea, R. Eddy, T.B. Shows, K. Philpott, A.L. Mellor, T.J. Knott, and J. Scott. 1986. cDNA sequence and chromosomal localization of human platelet-derived growth factor A-chain and its expression in tumour cell lines. *Nature* **320:** 695.

Browder, T.M., C.E. Dunbar, and A.W. Nienhuis. 1989. Private and public autocrine loops in neoplastic cells. *Cancer Cells* **1:** 9.

Clarke, M.F., E. Westin, D. Schmidt, S.F. Josephs, L. Ratner, F. Wong-Staal, R.C. Gallo, and M.S. Reitz. 1984. Transformation of NIH 3T3 cells by a human c-*sis* cDNA clone. *Nature* **308:** 464.

Connell, N.D. and J.G. Rheinwald. 1983. Regulation of the cytoskeleton in mesothelial cells: Reversible loss of keratin and increase in vimentin during rapid growth in culture. *Cell* **34:** 245.

Demetri, G.D., B.W. Zenzie, J.G. Rheinwald, and J.D. Griffin. 1989.

Expression of colony-stimulating factor genes by normal human mesothelial cells and human malignant mesothelioma cells lines in vitro. *Blood* **74**: 940.

Derynck, R., J.A. Jarrett, E.Y. Chen, and D.V. Goeddel. 1986. The murine transforming growth factor-β precursor. *J. Biol. Chem.* **261**: 4377.

Earp, H.S., J.R. Hepler, L.A. Petch, A. Miller, A.R. Berry, J. Harris, V.W. Raymond, B.K. McCune, L.W. Lee, J.W. Grisham, and T.K. Harden. 1988. Epidermal growth factor (EGF) and hormones stimulate phosphoinositide hydrolysis and increase EGF receptor protein synthesis and mRNA levels in rat liver epithelial cells. *J. Biol. Chem.* **263**: 13868.

Gabrielson, E.W., J.F. Lechner, B.I. Gerwin, M.A. LaVeck, and C.C. Harris. 1987. Growth factors for mesothelial and mesothelioma cells. *Chest* **91**: 71S.

Gerwin, B.I., J.F. Lechner, R.R. Reddel, A.B. Roberts, K.C. Robbins, E.W. Gabrielson, and C.C. Harris. 1987. Comparison of production of transforming growth factor-β and platelet-derived growth factor by normal human mesothelial cells and mesothelioma cell lines. *Cancer Res.* **47**: 6180.

Gerwin, B.I., C. Betsholtz, K. Linnainmaa, K. Pelin, R. Reddel, E. Gabrielson, M. Seddon, R. Greenwald, C.C. Harris, and J. Lechner. 1990. In vitro studies of human mesothelioma. In *Biological toxicology and carcinogenesis of respiratory epithelium* (ed. D.G. Thomasson and P. Nettesheim), p. 112. Hemisphere Publishing, Washington, D.C.

Gunning, P., P. Ponte, H. Okayama, J. Engel, H. Blau, and L. Kedes. 1983. Isolation and characterization of full-length cDNA clones for human α-, β- and γ-actin mRNAs: Skeletal but not cytoplasmic actins have an amino-terminal cystein that is subsequently removed. *Mol. Cell. Biol.* **3**: 787.

Jaurand, M.C. 1989. Particle-state carcinogenesis: A survey of recent studies on the mechanisms of action of fibers. *IARC Sci. Publ.* **90**: 54.

Jaurand, M.C., J.F. Bernaudin, A. Renier, H. Kaplan, and J. Bignon. 1981. Rat pleural mesothelial cells in culture. *In Vitro* **17**: 98.

LaRocca, P.J. and J.G. Rheinwald. 1985. Anchorage-independent growth of normal human mesothelial cells: A sensitive bioassay for EGF which discloses the absence of this factor in fetal calf serum. *In Vitro Cell. Dev. Biol.* **21**: 67.

Laveck, M.A., A.N.A. Somers, L.L. Moore, B.I. Gerwin, and J.F. Lechner. 1988. Dissimilar peptide growth factors can induce normal human mesothelial cell multiplication. *In Vitro Cell. Dev. Biol.* **24**: 1077.

Lee, D.C., T.M. Rose, N.R. Webb, and G.J. Todaro. 1985. Cloning and sequence analysis of a cDNA for rat transforming growth factor-α. *Nature* **313**: 489.

Roberts, A.B. and M.B. Sporn. 1986. Growth factors and transformation. *Cancer Surv.* **5:** 405.

Shimasaki, S., N. Emoto, A. Koba, M. Mercado, F. Shibata, K. Cooksey, A. Baird, and N. Lung. 1988. Complementary DNA cloning and sequencing of rat ovarian basic fibroblast growth factor and tissue distribution study of its mRNA. *Biochem. Biophys. Res. Commun.* **157:** 256.

Sporn, M.B. and A.B. Roberts. 1985. Autocrine growth factors and cancer. *Nature* **313:** 745.

Van der Meeren, A., G. Clement, J. Bignon, D. Baritault, and M.C. Jaurand. 1989. Production of growth factors by rat pleural mesothelial cells in vivo or in vitro transformed by chrysotile fibers. *NATO ASI Ser. Ser. H Cell Biol.* **30:** 133.

Van der Meeren, A., F. Levy, A. Renier, A. Katz, and M.C. Jaurand. 1990. Effect of epidermal growth factor on rat pleural mesothelial cell growth. *J. Cell Physiol.* **144:** 137.

Versnel, M.A., A. Hagemeijer, M.J. Bouts, T.H. van der Kwast, and K.C. Hoogsteden. 1988. Expression of c-*sis* (PDGF B-chain) and PDGF A-chain genes in ten human malignant mesothelioma cell lines derived from primary and metastatic tumors. *Oncogene* **2:** 601.

Yarden, Y., J.A. Escobedo, W.-J. Kuang, T.L. Yang-Feng, T.O. Daniel, P.M. Tremble, E.Y. Chen, M.E. Ando, R.N. Harkins, U. Francke, V.A. Fried, A. Ullrich, and L.T. Williams. 1986. Structure of the receptor for platelet-derived growth factors helps define a family of closely related growth factor receptors. *Nature* **323:** 226.

Role of Active Oxygen Species in Asbestos-induced Cytotoxicity, Cell Proliferation, and Carcinogenesis

B.T. Mossman and J.P. Marsh

Department of Pathology, University of Vermont College of Medicine
Burlington, Vermont 05405

INTRODUCTION

Inhalation of asbestos fibers was associated in the past work-place with the development of malignancies of the respiratory tract. Bronchogenic carcinoma, a cancer originating from the epithelial cells that line the air spaces or alveoli, is a tumor that predominates in asbestos workers who smoke (Mossman and Gee 1989; Mossman et al. 1990a). These tumors rarely occur in nonsmokers who have worked with asbestos. Meso-thelioma is a tumor developing in the visceral or parietal pleura of the lung. In contrast with bronchogenic carcinoma, the occurrence of malignant mesotheliomas in humans is un-related to smoking habits.

The mechanisms of induction and development of these two dissimilar tumors appear to be distinct. Asbestos appears to be a tumor promoter or cocarcinogen in the development of bronchogenic carcinoma, whereas it resembles a complete car-cinogen in the causation of mesothelioma (Mossman et al. 1990a). For example, in vitro exposure to asbestos results in chromosomal changes in mesothelial cells, but aneuploidy and DNA breakage are not observed in rodent or human tracheo-bronchial epithelial cells. However, mesothelial and tracheo-bronchial epithelial cells undergo alterations in proliferation, after exposure to asbestos, that may be important during the promotion state of carcinogenesis (Mossman et al. 1985; Moalli et al. 1987).

In inhalation models, asbestos causes a common sequence of events in the respiratory tract that precedes the develop-ment of disease (Mossman et al. 1990a). An initial inflammatory response, characterized by infiltration of alveolar macro-phages (AMs) into the air spaces and the accumulation of polymorphonuclear leukocytes (PMN) and lymphocytes, occurs before obvious lung injury and histopathologic changes (Pet-ruska et al. 1990). Both recruited and resident cells of the lung interact directly with inhaled asbestos and phagocytize fibers. Since longer, thinner (ca. >5 µm long) fibers of asbestos are more cytotoxic in vitro (Mossman et al. 1986) and more pathogenic than shorter fibers in the induction of mesotheli-oma in rodents (Stanton and Wrench 1972; Davis et al. 1986), we hypothesized that longer asbestos fibers caused elaboration of active oxygen species (AOS) from cells during incomplete phagocytosis. The geometry of the fiber also appears important to response. For example, both freshly isolated hamster and rat AMs release the AOS, superoxide (O_2^-) in a dosage-depen-dent manner when exposed to asbestos or nonasbestos fibers (defined as a >3:1 length-to-dia. ratio), such as glass and erionite, but particles (defined as a <3:1 length-to-dia. ratio) of similar chemical composition are less effective (Hansen and Mossman 1987). Moreover, long chrysotile asbestos fibers (>10 µm) in comparison with short fibers (<2 µm) cause greater release of O_2^- from these cell types (Mossman et al. 1989). In support of our hypothesis that AOS are important mediators of asbestos-induced toxicity, administration of anti-oxidant en-zymes to tracheal epithelial cells in vitro prevents cytotoxicity induced by crocidolite and long (>10 µm) chrysotile fibers (Mossman et al. 1986).

After exposure to crocidolite or chrysotile asbestos in vitro, a compensatory increase in antioxidant enzymes occurs in tracheal epithelial cells, although at high concentrations of as-bestos, this increase appears insufficient to protect the cell (Mossman et al. 1986). Presently, we are investigating the me-chanisms whereby asbestos fibers cause increases in anti-oxidant enzymes in lung cells both in vitro and after inhalation of asbestos. Preliminary data show that crocidolite asbestos causes increased steady-state mRNA levels of one or more antioxidant enzymes in the lung in a rat inhalation model of disease (Mossman et al. 1991). These experiments suggest that asbestos induces increased gene expression of enzymes involved in lung defense against minerals.

The objective of studies described here was to determine whether asbestos also influences gene expression of an enzyme involved in cell proliferation, a phenomenon that may be important during tumor promotion. In this regard, we have focused on ornithine decarboxylase (ODC) as a rate-limiting enzyme in the biosynthesis of polyamines. Polyamines are growth-regulatory molecules in cells that must be increased before cell division occurs and are causally implicated in tumor promotion. For example, the potency of the classical tumor promoter, 12-0-tetradecanoylphorbol-13-acetate (TPA), and chemically similar analogs is directly related to their ability to induce ODC in the mouse skin model of carcinogenesis (O'Brien 1976).

We have shown previously that both chrysotile and crocidolite asbestos induce ODC activity in hamster tracheal epithelial (HTE) cells in a manner similar to TPA (Landesman and Mossman 1982). Inhibitors of calcium transport and protein kinase C (PKC) inhibit asbestos-induced ODC activity in these cells (Marsh and Mossman 1988). In investigations presented here, we measured message levels of ODC in HTE cells after exposure to asbestos alone and in combination with antioxidant enzymes.

METHODS

Hamster tracheal epithelial cells. HTE cells are a diploid cell line isolated from the tracheal epithelium of a neonatal golden Syrian hamster (Mossman et al. 1980). Cells were used at passages <50 and maintained in Ham's F-12 medium supplemented with garamycin (100 µg/ml; M.A. Bioproducts, Walkersville, Maryland) and 10% fetal bovine serum (GIBCO, Grand Island, New York).

Asbestos. At confluency, cells were exposed for 4 hours to nontoxic concentrations of Union Internationale Contre le Cancer reference samples of crocidolite (0.64 µg/cm^2 dish) or Rhodesian chrysotile asbestos (0.32 µg/cm^2 dish) as described previously (Marsh and Mossman 1988). These concentrations of asbestos cause increases in ODC activity and increased incorporation of [³H]thymidine in HTE cells (Landesman and Mossman 1982).

Addition of antioxidants. Selected antioxidant enzymes that protect cells and tissues from asbestos-induced cell damage were used in these investigations (Mossman et al. 1986). They included a combination of the enzymes superoxide dismutase (SOD) (400 U/ml), which catalyzes the dismutation of O_2^- to H_2O_2, catalase (5600 U/ml), the enzyme responsible for the decomposition of H_2O_2 to O_2 and H_2O, and a nonenzymatic scavenger of OH·, mannitol (10 mM). Preliminary studies showed that antioxidants alone had no effect on ODC activity.

Isolation of RNA. Total cellular RNA was isolated from HTE cells by a single-extraction method using acid guanidinium thiocyanate, phenol, and chloroform (Chomczynski and Sacchi 1987). RNA was then denatured and fractionated by electrophoresis on a 1.0% agarose-formaldehyde gel. To ensure that an equal amount of RNA was present in each lane of the gel, RNA was quantified by UV absorption, reprecipitated, washed, and quantitated a second time before loading each lane with RNA (15 μg). RNA then was transferred to nitrocellulose, baked, and hybridized with heat-denatured oligo-labeled probe. ODC cDNA (pOD$_{48}$), cloned from a mouse lymphoma cell line, was the kind gift from Dr. P. Coffino (University of California) (McConlogue et al. 1984). A probe for 28S rRNA (pI19), obtained from Dr. K Cutroneo (Department of Biochemistry, University of Vermont), was used as a housekeeping probe. Blots were washed and visualized by exposure to Kodak X-Omat AR film at −70°C using intensifying screens.

RESULTS AND DISCUSSION

In our experiments, we used concentrations of asbestos that caused increases in ODC activity in HTE cells (Marsh and Mossman 1988). To determine whether increased ODC activity corresponded to increased steady-state levels of ODC mRNA, HTE cells were exposed for 4 hours to asbestos in the presence or absence of antioxidants. Results, as quantitated by densitometry, are shown in Figure 1. Autoradiographs of Northern

ODC mRNA DENSITOMETRIC ANALYSIS

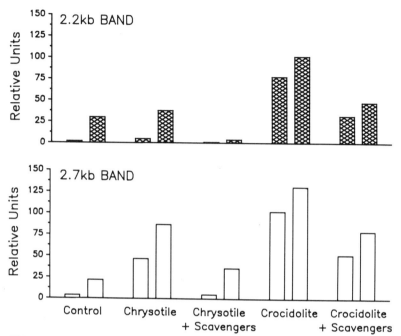

FIGURE 1 Northern blot analysis of mRNA for ODC after exposure of confluent HTE cells to chrysotile or crocidolite. Individual bars represent individual treatment groups (duplicate samples for experimental groups). RNA was isolated from two pooled 100-mm petri dishes/group, and 15 µg of RNA was fractionated in an agarose-formaldehyde gel, blotted onto nitrocellulose, and hybridized to ^{32}P-oligo-labeled pOD_{48} DNA. RNA bands containing ODC mRNAs were visualized by exposing Kodak X-Omat AR film to the washed blot (–70°C) with intensifying screens. Steady-state mRNA levels were quantitated using a Betagen apparatus.

blots in these experiments showed two species of mRNA with major bands at approximately 2.2 kb and 2.7 kb, which is comparable to the findings of Hickok et al. (1986) and Pohjanpelto et al. (1985). A dose-dependent induction of the mRNAs for ODC, corresponding to the magnitude of enzyme activation (Marsh and Mossman 1991) was seen after addition of either chrysotile or crocidolite. Amounts of mRNA were reduced after simultaneous addition of a mix of the antioxidants, SOD, catalase, and mannitol. Northern blot analysis, using the 28S housekeeping probe (PI19), confirmed that all lanes were loaded equally. For each lane probed with PI19, an average of 71.5 ± 2.8 cpm was obtained (Betascope blot analyzer, Betagen Corp., Waltham, Massachusetts).

The data here suggest that asbestos-stimulated induction of ODC gene expression involves an AOS-generating mechanism. This observation supports our results using a rodent inhalation model of disease. In these investigations, long-term administration of polyethylene-glycol (PEG)-conjugated catalase ameliorated inflammatory and fibrotic responses in rats exposed to crocidolite (Mossman et al. 1990c).

Asbestos may generate AOS either extracellularly or intracellularly by several mechanisms. For example, iron on the fiber surface may drive redox reactions, such as the Haber-Weiss reaction that ultimately produces OH· (Weitzman and Graceffa 1984; Zalma et al. 1988). This phenomenon may occur in the absence of fiber-cell interactions. Alternatively, asbestos, after interaction with the plasma membrane, may stimulate the nicotinamideadenine dinucleotide phosphate oxidase of phagocytic cells, such as macrophages and neutrophils, resulting in a "respiratory burst" and generation of O_2^- (Hansen and Mossman 1987).

ODC activation triggered by asbestos (Landesman and Mossman 1982) or oxidants (Marsh and Mossman 1991) in HTE cells leads to subsequent proliferative changes, as measured by incorporation of a radiolabeled nucleotide into DNA. Both asbestos (Mossman et al. 1980) and generation of AOS by the chemical generation system of xanthine and xanthine oxidase result in the development of hyperplasia and squamous metaplasia in hamster tracheal organ cultures (Mossman et al. 1990b; Radosevich and Weitzman 1989). These observations indicate a direct relationship between AOS, proliferation, and tumor promotion in epithelial cells of the respiratory tract.

A hypothetical schema for elaboration of AOS by asbestos is illustrated in Figure 2. In this scenario of events, fibers may interact with cells of the immune system that produce AOS,

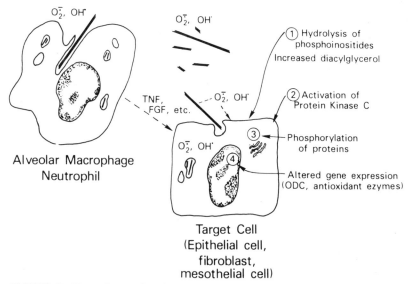

FIGURE 2 Hypothetical scheme illustrating several pathways for the elaboration of AOS by asbestos.

including O_2^- and OH·. This generation may be exacerbated after cell interaction with long fibers that are incompletely phagocytized. Cytokines, such as tumor necrosis factor-α or fibroblast growth factor released from activated AMs, might also cause the production of AOS from target cells of the lung, as has been reported in human skin fibroblasts (Meier et al. 1989). Other possible mechanisms of production of AOS by asbestos include redox reactions occurring on the fiber surface or interaction of fibers directly with target cells.

Cell-signaling mechanisms governing ODC activation by soluble tumor promoters, such as TPA and insoluble mineral fibers, may be similar. For example, exposure of HTE cells to asbestos in vitro causes hydrolysis of phosphoinositides and the formation of diacylglycerol (Sesko et al. 1990), whereas TPA mimics diacylglycerol by binding to and activating its cellular receptor, PKC (for review, see Blumberg 1988). Activation of PKC appears essential to both TPA- (Verma et al. 1986) and asbestos-stimulated ODC induction (Marsh and Mossman 1988). Thus, a plausible sequence of signaling events may involve asbestos-induced phosphoinositide hydrolysis, producing diacylglycerol, which then activates PKC. In turn, PKC through altered protein phosphorylation may induce ODC and lead to altered proliferation during the process of tumor promotion. Our experiments suggest that induction of ODC by asbestos occurs at the level of transcription analogous to events documented after application of TPA to mouse skin (Gilmour et al. 1987). Thus, results here and from our earlier investigations documenting increased gene expression of antioxidant enzymes in lung cells exposed to asbestos in vivo suggest that this fibrous mineral induces genes involved in both cell proliferation and lung defense.

ACKNOWLEDGMENTS

We acknowledge the assistance of Judith Kessler and Laurie Sabens in the preparation of this manuscript and grant support from National Heart, Lung, and Blood Institute (HL-396469, SCOR HL-14212).

REFERENCES

Blumberg, P.M. 1988. Protein kinase C as the receptor for the phorbol ester tumor promoters: Sixth Rhoads Memorial Award Lecture. *Cancer Res.* **48**: 1.

Chomczynski, P. and N. Sacchi. 1987. Single-step method of RNA isolation by acid guanidinium thiocyanate-phenol-chloroform extraction. *Anal. Biochem.* **162**: 156.

Davis, J.M.G., J. Addison, R.E. Bolton, K. Donaldson, A.D. Jones, and T. Smith. 1986. The pathogenicity of long versus short fibre samples of amosite asbestos administered to rats by inhalation and intraperitoneal injection. *Br. J. Exp. Pathol.* **67**: 415.

Gilmour, S.K., A.K. Verma, T. Madara, and T.G. O'Brien. 1987. Regulation of ornithine decarboxylase gene expression in mouse epidermis and epidermal tumors during two-stage tumorigenesis. *Cancer Res.* **47**: 1221.

Hansen, K. and B.T. Mossman. 1987. Generation of superoxide (O_2^- from aveolar macrophages exposed to asbestiform and nonfibrous particles. *Cancer Res.* **47**: 1681.

Hickok, N.J., P.J. Seppänen, K.K. Kontula, P.A. Jänne, C.W. Bardin, and O.A. Jänne. 1986. Two ornithine decarboxylase mRNA species in mouse kidney arise from size heterogeneity at their 3′ termini. *Proc. Natl. Acad. Sci.* **83**: 594.

Landesman, J.M. and B.T. Mossman. 1982. Induction of ornithine decarboxylase in hamster tracheal epithelial cells exposed to asbestos and 12-0-tetradecanoylphorbol-13-acetate. *Cancer Res.* **42:** 3669.

Marsh, J.P. and B.T. Mossman. 1988. Mechanisms of induction of ornithine decarboxylase activity in tracheal epithelial cells by asbestiform minerals. *Cancer Res.* **48:** 709.

――――. 1991. Role of asbestos and active oxygen species in activation and expression of ornithine decarboxylase in hamster tracheal epithelial cells. *Cancer Res.* (in press).

McConlogue, L., M. Gupta, L. Wu, and P. Coffino. 1984. Molecular cloning and expression of the mouse ornithine decarboxylase gene. *Proc. Natl. Acad. Sci.* **81:** 540.

Meier, B., H.H. Radeke, S. Selle, M. Younes, H. Sies, K. Resch, and G.G. Habermehl. 1989. Human fibroblasts release reactive oxygen species in response to interleukin-1 or tumour necrosis factor-α. *Biochem. J.* **263:** 539.

Moalli, P.A., J.L. MacDonald, L.A. Goodglick, and A.B. Kane. 1987. Acute injury and regeneration of the mesothelium in response to asbestos fibers. *Am. J. Pathol.* **128:** 426.

Mossman, B.T. and J.B.L. Gee. 1989. Medical progress. Asbestos-associated disease. *N. Engl. J. Med.* **320:** 1721.

Mossman, B.T., G.S. Cameron, and L.P. Yotti. 1985. Cocarcinogenic and tumor promoting properties of asbestos and other minerals in tracheobronchial epithelium. *Carcinog. Compr. Surv.* **8:** 217.

Mossman, B.T., J.P. Marsh, and M.A. Shatos. 1986. Alteration of superoxide dismutase activity in tracheal epithelial cells by asbestos and inhibition of cytotoxicity by antioxidants. *Lab. Invest.* **54:** 204.

Mossman, B.T., E.B. Ezerman, K.B. Adler, and J.E. Craighead. 1980. Isolation and spontaneous transformation of hamster tracheal epithelial cells. *Cancer Res.* **40:** 4403.

Mossman, B.T., J. Bignon, M. Corn, J.B.L. Gee, and A. Seaton. 1990a. Asbestos: Scientific developments and implications for public policy. *Science* **247:** 294.

Mossman, B.T., J.P. Marsh, R. Dantona, M. Bergeron, and A. Senior. 1990b. Involvement of active oxygen species (AOS) in injury, repair and proliferation of tracheobronchial epithelial cells after exposure to asbestos fibers. In *Biology, toxicology and carcinogenesis of respiratory epithelium* (ed. D.G. Thomassen and P. Nettesheim), p. 145. Hemisphere Publication, New York.

Mossman, B.T., K. Hansen, J.P. Marsh, M.E. Brew, S. Hill, M. Bergeron, and J. Petruska. 1989. Mechanisms of fibre-induced superoxide release from alveolar macrophages and induction of superoxide dismutase in the lungs of rats inhaling crocidolite. *IARC Publ.* **90:** 81.

Mossman, B.T., Y.M.W. Janssen, J.P. Marsh, M. Manohar, M. Garrone, S. Shull, and D. Hemenway. 1991. Antioxidant defense mechanisms in asbestos-induced lung disease. *J. Aerosol Med.* (in press).

Mossman, B.T., J.P. Marsh, A. Sesko, S. Hill, M.A. Shatos, J. Doherty, J. Petruska, K.B. Adler, D. Hemenway, R. Mickey, P. Vacek, and E. Kagan. 1990c. Inhibition of lung injury, inflammation and interstitial pulmonary fibrosis by polyethylene glycol-conjugated catalase in a rapid inhalation model of asbestosis. *Am. Rev. Respir. Dis.* **141:** 1266.

O'Brien, T.G. 1976. The induction of ornithine decarboxylase as an early, possibly obligatory, event in mouse skin carcinogenesis. *Cancer Res.* **36:** 2644.

Petruska, J.M., J. Marsh, M. Bergeron, and B.T. Mossman. 1990. Brief inhalation of asbestos compromises superoxide production in cells from bronchoalveolar lavage. *Am. J. Respir. Cell Mol. Biol.* **2:** 129.

Pohjanpelto, P., E. Hölttä, and O. Jänne, S. Knuutila, and K. Hlitalo. 1985. Amplification of ornithine decarboxylase gene in response to polyamine deprivation in Chinese hamster ovary cells. *J. Biol. Chem.* **260:** 8532.

Radosevich, C.A. and S.A. Weitzman. 1989. Hydrogen peroxide induces squamous metaplasia in a hamster tracheal organ explant culture model. *Carcinogenesis* **10:** 1943.

Sesko, A., M. Cabot, and B.T. Mossman. 1990. Hydrolysis of phosphoinositides precedes cellular proliferation in asbestos-stimulated tracheobronchial epithelial cells. *Proc. Natl. Acad. Sci.* **87:** 7385.

Stanton, M.F. and C. Wrench. 1972. Mechanisms of mesothelioma induction with asbestos and fibrous glass. *J. Natl. Cancer Inst.* **48:** 797.

Verma, A.K., R.C. Pong, and D. Erikson. 1986. Involvement of protein kinase C activation in ornithine decarboxylase gene expression in primary cultures of newborn mouse epidermal cells and in skin tumor promotion by 12-0-tetradecanoylphorbol-13-acetate. *Cancer Res.* **46:** 6149.

Weitzman, S.A. and P. Graceffa. 1984. Asbestos catalyzes hydroxyl and superoxide radical generation from hydrogen peroxide. *Arch. Biochem. Biophys.* **228:** 373.

Zalma, R., L. Bonneau, M.C. Jaurand, J. Guignard, and H. Pezerat. 1988. Formation of oxy-radicals by oxygen reduction arising from the surface activity of asbestos. *Can. J. Chem.* **65:** 2338.

Radiation and Asbestos Fibers: Interaction and Mechanisms

T.K. Hei, C.Q. Piao, and Z.Y. He

Center for Radiological Research
Columbia University College of Physicians & Surgeons
New York, New York 10032

INTRODUCTION

The carcinogenicity of asbestos fibers has been well established in both humans and experimental animals (Harrington 1976). Furthermore, cigarette smoking can enhance the lung cancer incidence among asbestos workers in a synergistic fashion (Selikoff et al. 1968). Apart from the numerous chemicals including various polycyclic aromatic hydrocarbons that have been identified in cigarette smoke (Hoffmann et al. 1974), cigarettes also contain trace amounts of ^{210}P, an α-emitting radionucleotide (Radford and Hunt 1964). It is not known for certain whether specific chemicals or the high-linear-energy-transfer (LET) α-particles are the important factor in carcinogenesis caused by cigarettes and its enhancement by asbestos. It has been estimated that an average smoker who smokes two packs of cigarettes a day for 25 years would receive 75 cGy of these densely ionizing particles from smoking alone. Epidemiological data have also suggested a synergistic interaction between radiation and cigarette smoke in the induction of lung cancer among uranium miners (Bair 1970). The importance of these high-LET α-particles has recently been reemphasized with the realization that environmental radon represents the largest source of natural background radiation to which the United States population is exposed (NCRP Report 1984).

The mechanism(s) by which asbestos fibers produce malignancy is not entirely clear at present. Various in vivo and in vitro studies, however, have suggested that fiber dimensions, not chemical contaminants the native fiber may have con-

Cellular and Molecular Aspects of Fiber Carcinogenesis

tained, are crucial to the carcinogenicity of the fibers, since leaching does not affect carcinogenic potential (Wagner and Berry 1969; Stanton et al. 1977; Hei et al. 1985). Although chromosomal changes and aneuploidy have been demonstrated in several studies, other genotoxic endpoints used to measure the biological effects of asbestos are thus far inconsistent (Daniel 1983). The implication that risk of developing asbestos-related diseases may extend beyond that of an occupational hazard suggests the importance of a long-term, low-dosage exposure to a large number of people. The fact that radiation, cigarette smoke, and asbestos, three main environmental carcinogens, can interact in a synergistic fashion in cancer induction highlights the complexity in risk estimation and emphasizes the urgent need for basic research on the mechanisms of their interaction.

Biological Effects of High- versus Low-LET Radiations

The He^3 ions used in these studies have a LET value of 120 keV/μm and are similar to the energy spectrum of radon α-particles. Figure 1a shows the survival and transformation data for gamma-rays and high-LET He^3 ions. The cell survival curve for gamma-rays has a broad initial shoulder, whereas the curve for He^3 ions approximates closely to an exponential function of dose, indicating single-hit kinetics, i.e., the cell is killed by the traversal of a single particle. On the basis of microdosimetric analysis, it has been estimated that at D_0, which is a dose that corresponds to a survival fraction of 37%, about 14 particles traverse the nucleus of each cell killed. Although one particle is sufficient to kill the cell, on average about 13 particles traverse the cell without killing it for every one "hit" that does! This may explain the high-oncogenic-transforming-potential of high-LET radiations.

The C3H/10T1/2 cells used were originally cloned and characterized by Reznikoff et al. (1973). These cells exhibit contact inhibition of growth under normal culture conditions. When treated with physical or chemical carcinogens, isolated foci appear consisting of morphologically altered cells. These cells are anchorage independent and produce fibrosarcomas on inoculation into syngeneic animals. The transformation in-

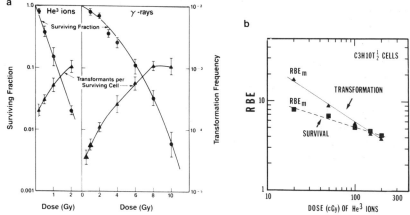

FIGURE 1 (a) Cell survival and oncogenic transformation incidence as a function of dose for He^3 ions and gamma-rays. The He^3 ions have LET values comparable with the α-particles emitted by radon daughter products. Data are compiled from four to five experiments. Bars, ± S.E.M. (b) RBE as a function of dose for cell lethality and oncogenic transformation. RBE is defined as the ratio of doses of low/ high-LET radiations to achieve similar biological effects. Calculated from the data of Fig. 1a. (Reprinted, with permission, from Hall et al. 1989.)

cidence induced by both He^3 ions and gamma-rays is shown in Figure 1a. The incidence is expressed as transformants per surviving cell. For both types of radiation, transformation incidence increases with dose, and for gamma-rays, the frequency shows a plateau at about 8 Gy. Figure 1b is a plot of the relative biological effectiveness (RBE) as a function of dose calculated from the data of Figure 1a for both cell survival and transformation. For high-LET radiation, the RBE for cellular transformation at low doses is substantially higher than for cell killing. With increasing doses, the killing effect becomes more critical, and the RBE for transformation decreases gradually.

Interaction between Asbestos Fibers and Low-LET Radiation

Various in vitro studies have shown that, in addition to the in vivo targets of asbestos fibers (macrophages and mesothelial cells), fibroblasts of different origins, including C3H/10T1/2 and hamster embryo cells, can phagocytize the fibers in a dose-dependent manner (Beck 1976; Hei et al. 1987). Both crocidolite and amosite fibers induce a dose-dependent toxicity in C3H/10T1/2 cells, and leaching the fibers with organic solvent does not alter the toxicity at low-fiber concentrations (Hei et al. 1985). Combined treatments of fibers and gamma-irradiation result in a survival that is additive in nature. No difference between unleached and acid-leached fibers is found. The interaction between different physical and chemical agents in the production of transformation is a topic of importance in risk estimate for radiation protection. Figure 2 shows

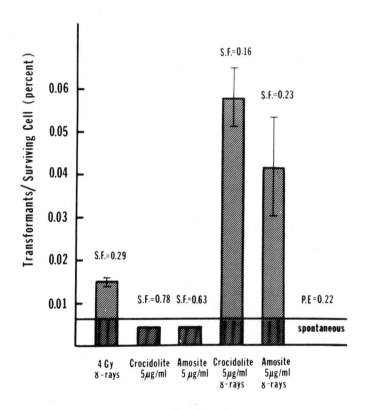

Treatments

FIGURE 2 Transformation incidence in C3H/10T1/2 cells treated with a 5 μg/ml dose of either crocidolite or amosite fibers for 24 hr with or without a concurrent 4 Gy dose of ^{137}Cs gamma-rays. Darker shaded area depicts spontaneous frequency. (S.F.) Surviving fraction; (P.E.) plating efficiency. (Drawn using data from Hei et al. 1984.)

the effects of gamma-irradiation combined with two types of asbestos fibers on the transformation incidence in C3H/10T1/2 cells. Although asbestos fibers at a concentration that resulted in only moderate cell killing were nononcogenic by themselves, they were found to enhance the transforming potential of gamma-rays in a more than additive fashion. Furthermore, leaching the fibers did not affect this synergistic interaction with gamma-irradiation. Clearly, this cocarcinogenic effect of the fiber for radiation-induced transformation cannot be attributed to leachable contaminants and must therefore reflect a property of the fibers themselves.

Interaction of Asbestos Fibers with Radon-simulated α-Particles

The facts that asbestos fibers and cigarette smoking interact in a synergistic fashion in lung cancer induction among asbestos workers and that cigarette smoke contains picocurie quantities of ^{210}P radionucleotide suggest the possible interaction between α-particles and asbestos. The effects of asbestos fibers in concert with densely ionizing particles on oncogenic transformation incidence were examined, and the results are shown in Figure 3. The transformation frequency resulting from a 24-hour pretreatment with 5 µg/ml crocidolite fibers or a dose of 66 cGy He^3 ions is presented. As shown previously with low-LET radiation, crocidolite fibers at concentrations that result in only moderate cell killing induced transformation frequencies indistinguishable from the spontaneous rate. However, cells pretreated with crocidolite fibers for 24 hours and subsequently irradiated with α-particles exhibited a significantly higher-transformation incidence than those receiving radiation alone. The combination of asbestos fibers and high-LET α-particles produces a transformation incidence higher than the sum of the two agents alone. This apparent supra-additivity has implications for the possible interaction of radon and asbestos in the environment and possibly for combinations of other environmental pollutants.

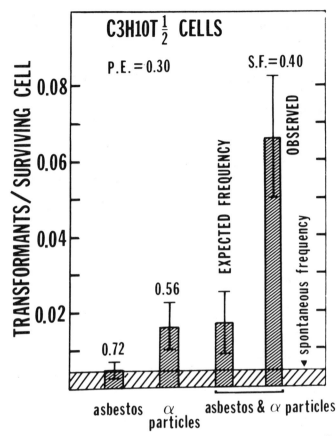

FIGURE 3 Transformation incidence in C3H/10T1/2 cells treated with a 5 μg/ml dose of crocidolite fibers and He[3] ions, delivered either alone or in combination. There is apparent supra-additivity in the interaction when asbestos and high-LET particles are delivered together. (Reprinted, with permission, from Hei 1989.)

Mechanisms of Radiation-Fiber Interaction: Role of Oxygen Radicals

Stanton's theory of fiber carcinogenesis (Stanton et al. 1977) suggests a positive correlation between the dimension of asbestos fibers and their carcinogenic potential. Fibers that are long and thin are more carcinogenic than fibers that are short and thick. The importance of fiber-cell interaction is obvious when considering the observation that fibers longer than 25 μm are generally not completely phagocytized by cells, and common channels have been demonstrated between the extracellular and intracellular spaces at the site of interaction (Beck 1976).

The involvement of superoxide anions in asbestos-induced cytotoxicity has been suggested previously (Hansen and Mossman 1987). The radical scavenging enzyme, superoxide dismutase (SOD), has been shown to protect against the in vitro cytotoxicity of asbestos fibers (Mossman et al. 1986). Are oxyradicals mechanistically involved in the radiation-fiber interaction? Figure 4 shows the effects of SOD and catalase on the oncogenic-transforming potential resulting from a fiber-radiation interaction in C3H/10T1/2 cells. Although addition of either SOD or catalase to the culture medium had little or no effect on the cytotoxicity of the fibers, addition of SOD ob-

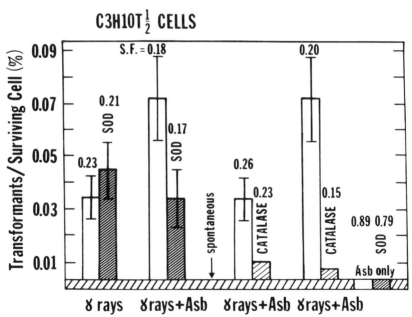

FIGURE 4 Transformation incidence in C3H/10T1/2 cells produced by the various treatment in either the presence (closed bars) or the absence (open bars) of either SOD or catalase. Results are compiled from three experiments. Bars, ± S.E.M. (S.F.) Surviving fraction. (Reprinted, with permission, from Hei 1989.)

literated the supra-additive oncogenic transforming response characteristic of the radiation-fiber interaction to a level comparable with that of radiation alone. Similar results were also obtained with catalase, although this might be due to its suppressive effects on the expression of radiation-induced transformants. The discrepancy in the SOD data between the two studies may very likely be due to differences in the doses of asbestos and SOD that were used and the experimental design.

Pursuing the Mechanisms of Radiation-Fiber Interaction: Asbestos Fibers as Mutagens

The fact that oxygen-scavenging enzymes can obliterate the supra-additive effect of a combined gamma-ray and asbestos fiber treatment on transformation induction in C3H/10T1/2 cells suggests the importance of oxyradicals in such interactions. Various studies have implicated reactive oxygen species in the induction of gene mutations in bacteria and mammalian cells (Phillips et al. 1984). In addition, oxyradicals have also been linked directly to various in vivo and in vitro effects of asbestos fibers (Mossman et al. 1986). Hence, if oxyradicals are mechanistically involved in fiber carcinogenesis, as postulated, one would expect the fibers to be mutagenic. Data available for genotoxicity of the fibers, however, are not consistent. Although several types of asbestos fibers have been shown to induce chromosomal aberration in both rodent and human cells (Sincock et al. 1982; Lechner et al. 1985), reports on mutagenesis due to asbestos have largely been negative. Huang et al. (1978) reported the only positive mutagenic studies of asbestos fibers using Chinese hamster lung cells at the hypoxanthine-guanine phosphoribosyltransferase (HGPRT) locus with 6-thioguanine as the selective agent. Although the use of gene markers, such as the HGPRT, located on essential monosomic chromosomes provides an accurate and convenient measurement for agents that induce small gene mutations, chromosomal mutations, such as large deletions and chromosomal nondisjunction, can be underestimated if they extend into vital genes that result in the cell's death. The AL human-hamster hybrid cells, developed by Puck et al. (1971), contain a single copy of human chromosome 11 in addition to the standard set of hamster genomes. Several cell-surface antigenic markers have been identified on these cells and have been regionally mapped on the human chromosome. By the use of appropriate antibodies, mutations can be scored in the human chromosome with great specificity and quantification (Waldren et al. 1979; Hei et al. 1988). Since this chromosome is not vital to the AL cells, the entire chromosome can be used as a target for mutagenic events, thereby enhancing the sensitivity of the assay system. This provides a significant advantage over the use of conventional HGPRT as a mutation indicator.

Wild-type AL cells contain the surface antigen markers a_1 and a_2. The a_1 and a_2 markers are on opposite arms of the human chromosome. a_1 has been regionally mapped on the short arm at 11p13, whereas a_2 is located on the long arm at 11q13–11qter. In the presence of complement and specific antiserum against either a_1 or a_2 antigens, wild-type AL cells are lysed, whereas mutated cells that have lost the marker antigens survive (Hei et al. 1988). Figure 5 shows mutation induction by graded doses of crocidolite fibers in AL cells at either the a_1 or HGPRT locus within the same treated population. The frequencies were expressed as the number of induced mutants (observed-background) per 10^5 survivors. Consistent with several previous findings, results of the present studies showed no definite pattern in the dose-response relationship for mutant yield at the HGPRT locus through the range of concentrations examined. Although the absolute number of induced mutants at each concentration examined was not zero, there was no statistically significant difference in mutation between the highest and lowest doses studied. In contrast, crocidolite fibers induced dose-dependent mutagenesis at the a_1 locus from the same treated population. At the lowest fiber concentration examined (2.5 μg/ml), although crocidolite fibers induced a mutation frequency that was indistinguishable from the spontaneous level at the HGPRT locus, the same fibers induced a mutant fraction that was at least 50-fold higher at the a_1 locus.

Preliminary data on the analysis of DNA from the asbestos induced HGPRT⁻ mutants using a cDNA probe for the hamster gene (pHPT12) show mostly major deletions of the HGPRT se-

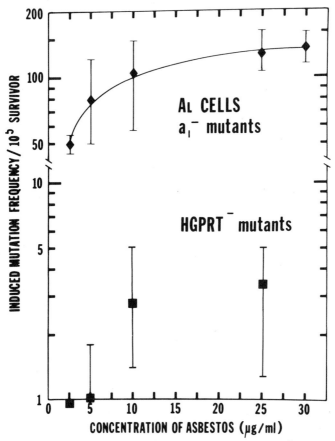

FIGURE 5 Induced mutation frequencies per 10^5 survivors at either the a_1 (diamonds) or the HGPRT (squares) loci in AL cells treated with graded doses of crocidolite asbestos fibers for 24 hr. Data are compiled from four to five experiments. Bars, ± S.E.M.

quence. The results so far suggest that crocidolite fibers (1) may be mutagenic and (2) that most of the genetic damage induced by the fibers are likely to be deletions. The fact that earlier studies failed to detect mutation by asbestos fibers at the HGPRT locus may be a consequence of large gene deletions that is not compatible with the survival of the 6-thioguanine-resistant mutants. Furthermore, the deletion type of damage induced by asbestos fibers is in agreement with the proposed oxyradical mechanism of fiber carcinogenesis, since recent studies using the polymerase chain reaction technique have suggested that reactive oxygen species induce mostly deletion mutations in mammalian cells (Hsie et al. 1990).

CONCLUDING REMARKS

It is apparent from the studies summarized here that radiation can interact with asbestos fibers in a supra-additive fashion, an observation that has been suggested from earlier human epidemiological studies on lung cancer incidence among uranium miners and asbestos workers who also smoke. Studies undertaken to elucidate the cellular and molecular mechanism(s) of the fiber-radiation interaction have demonstrated that oxyradicals may be important intermediates in the observed synergistic interaction. This finding is not unexpected because (1) ionizing radiations involve free-radical mechanisms and (2) various in vitro and in vivo studies have implicated the importance of oxygen radicals in the fibrogenic and, possibly, the carcinogenic effects of asbestos fibers, as well.

The involvement of oxyradicals, however, suggests that asbestos fibers might also be mutagenic, since most radical species have been found to be mutagens not only in the Ames's bacterial test, but in several mammalian gene loci, as well. The fact that asbestos has never been shown to be mutagenic in bacterial assay systems highlights the importance of fiber-cell interaction. Cells that do not take up the fibers will not undergo the "metabolic burst" associated with production of radical. It should be cautioned that many cytotoxic effects of mineral fibers may simply be attributable to their surface charge, since metal chelating agents have been shown to prevent hemolysis and reduce in vitro cytotoxicity. Recent studies using asbestos and nonasbestos fibers, however, have shown that chromosomal damages through physical disruption of the mitotic spindles may be important in aneuploidy induction and fiber carcinogenesis.

The AL mutation assay system, because of the extra human chromosome the cells contain, can score genetic damages ranging from small deletions to translocations of the entire chromosome. The mutation data presented here suggest that crocidolite fibers may not be an efficient inducer of point mutation and that most genetic damages induced by the fibers are deletions. By examining the mutational events at both the HGPRT and the human chromosome 11 within the AL cell system, a spectrum of genetic events induced by radiation and asbestos fibers can be quantitated. Such studies are currently underway.

ACKNOWLEDGMENTS

The authors thank Dr. Howard Lieberman for critical reading of the manuscript. This investigation was supported in part by National Cancer Institute grant CA-12536 and by Columbia University Biomedical Research Support grant RR05395-24.

REFERENCES

Bair, W.J. 1970. Inhalation of radionucleotides and carcinogenesis. In *Inhalation carcinogenesis* (ed. M.G. Hanna et al.), p. 77. U.S. Atomic Energy Commission, Washington, D.C.

Beck, E.J. 1976. Interaction between fibrous dust and cells in vitro. *Ann. Anat. Pathol.* **21:** 227.

Daniel, F.B. 1983. In vitro assessment of asbestos genotoxicity. *Environ. Health Perspect.* **53:** 163.

Hall, E.J., T.K. Hei, and C.Q. Piao. 1989. Transformation by simulated radon daughter alpha particles: Interaction with asbestos and modulation by tumor promoters. In *Cell transformation and radiation-induced cancer* (ed. K.H. Chadwick, et al.), p. 293. Adam Hilger, England.

Hanson, K. and B. Mossman. 1987. Generation of superoxide from alveoler macrophages, exposed to asbestoiforms and non-fibrous particles. *Cancer Res.* **47:** 1681.

Harrington, J.S. 1976. The biological effects of mineral fibres. *Anna. Anat. Pathol.* **21:** 155.

Hei, T.K. 1989. Oncogenic transformation by asbestos fibers and radon-simulate alpha particles. *NATO ASI Ser. Ser. H Cell Biol.* **30:** 389.

Hei, T.K. and S. Kushner. 1987. Radiation and asbestos fibers: Interaction and possible mechanism. In *Anticarcinogenesis and radiation protection* (ed. P. Cerutti et al.), p. 345. Plenum Press, New York.

Hei, T.K., E.J. Hall, and R.S. Osmak. 1984. Asbestos, radiation and oncogenic transformation. *Br. J. Cancer.* **50:** 717.

Hei, T.K., E.J. Hall, and C.A. Waldren. 1988. Mutation induction by neutrons as determined by an antibody complement mediated cell lysate system. I. Experimental observations. *Radiat. Res.* **115:** 281.

Hei, T.K., C.R. Geard, R.S. Osmak, and M. Travisano. 1985. Correlation of in vitro gentoxicity and oncogenicity induced by radiation and asbestos fibres. *Br. J. Cancer* **52:** 591.

Hoffmann, D., G. Rathkamp, and Y. Liu. 1974. On the isolation and identification of volatile and non-volatile *N*-nitrosamines and hydrazines in cigarette smoke. *IARC Monogr. Eval. Carcinog. Risk Chem. Hum.* **9:** 159.

Hsie, A.W., Z. Xu, Y. Yu, M.A. Sognier, and P. Hrelia. 1990. Molecular analysis of reactive oxygen species induced mammalian gene mutation. *Teratog. Carcinog. Mutagen* **10:** 155.

Huang, S.L., D. Saggioro, H. Michelmann, and H. Malling. 1978. Genetic effects of crocidolite asbestos in Chinese hamster lung cells. *Mutat. Res.* **57:** 225.

Lechner, J.F, T. Tokiwa, M. LaVeck, W.F. Benedict, S. Bankschlegel, H. Yeager, J.A. Barnegee, and C.C. Harris. 1985. Asbestos associated chromosomal changes in human mesothelial cells. *Proc. Natl. Acad. Sci.* **82:** 3884.

Mossman, B.T., J.P. Marsh, and M.A. Shatos. 1986. Alteration of superoxide dismutase activity in tracheal epithelial cells by asbestos and induction of cytotoxicity by antioxidants. *Lab. Invest.* **54:** 204.

NCRP Report. 1984. Evaluation of occupational and environmental exposures to radon and radon daughters in the U.S., report 79. National Council on Radiation Protection and Measurement, Washington, D.C.

Phillips, B.J., T. James, and D. Anderson. 1984. Genetic damages in CHO cells exposed to enzymatically generated active oxygen species. *Mutat. Res.* **126:** 265.

Puck, T.T., P. Wuchier, C. Jones, and F.T. Kao. 1971. Genetics of somatic mammalian cells: Lethal antigens and genetic markers for study of human linkage groups. *Proc. Natl. Acad. Sci.* **68:** 3102.

Radford, E. and V. Hunt. 1964. Polonium-210: A volatile radioelement in cigarettes. *Science* **143:** 247.

Reznikoff, K., J.S. Bertram, D.W. Brankow, and C. Heidelberger. 1973. Quantitative and qualitative studies on chemical transformation on cloned C_3H mouse embryo cells sensitive to post confluence inhibition of cell division. *Cancer Res.* **33:** 3239.

Selikoff, I.J., E.C. Hammond, and J. Churg. 1968. Asbestos exposure, smoking and neoplasia. *J. Am. Med. Assoc.* **204:** 104.

Sincock, A.M., J.D. Delhanty, and G.A. Casey. 1982. A comparison of the cytogenetic response to asbestos and glass fiber in CHO cell lines. *Mutat. Res.* **101:** 257.

Stanton, M.F., M. Layard, and A. Tegeris. 1977. Carcinogenesis of fibrous glass: Pleural response in the rat in relation to the fiber dimension. *J. Natl. Acad. Sci.* **58:** 587.

Wagner, J.C. and G. Berry. 1969. Mesothelioma in rats following inoculation with asbestos. *Br. J. Cancer* **23:** 567.

Waldren, C., C. Jones, and T.T. Puck. 1976. A measurement of mutagenesis in mammalian cells. *Proc. Natl. Acad. Sci.* **76:** 1358.

Use of Animal Models to Study Man-made Fiber Carcinogenesis

T.W. Hesterberg,[1] V. Vu,[2] G.R. Chase,[1]
E.E. McConnell,[3] W.B. Bunn,[1] and R. Anderson[1]

[1]Manville Technical Center, Littleton, Colorado 80127
[2]Office of Toxic Substances, U.S. Environmental Protection Agency
Washington, D.C. 20460
[3]Raleigh, North Carolina 27613

INTRODUCTION

The attributes of the dose reaching the target tissue are crucial in the assessment of protocols to study the toxicity of any material. The study of fiber carcinogenesis poses some distinctive challenges to achieve that end. In particular, it is necessary to size most fibers to the animal model of choice. Adequately sized fibers can then be used to attain desired doses by physiological routes, thus overcoming the limitations of other exposure methodologies.

There is a natural concern about the safety of any material that has the potential to give off particles or vapors that can be inhaled and/or ingested. There is a heightened awareness for all such fiber materials, and for that reason, there have been and continues to be many experimental and epidemiological studies dealing with both naturally occurring and man-made fibers.

Occupational cohort studies clearly show increased risks of lung cancer, mesothelioma, and nonmalignant respiratory disease associated with the inhalation of naturally occurring mineral fibers. The magnitude of the risks appear to vary by fiber type, occupational use, and lifestyle, e.g., cigarette smoking. Those pathogenic effects of mineral fibers are attributed, in general, to their fibrous nature. The concern for other fibers comes from the finding that many of those fibers also induce the same diseases in some experimental models. In particular, the pioneering work of Stanton (Stanton and Wrench 1972; Stanton et al. 1977, 1981) showed that by directly implanting fibers of similar size into the pleura of rats, thereby bypassing the natural route of exposure, mesotheliomas were produced. However, it is clear that although dimension is not the sole determinant of the toxicity of fibers, it may be one of the most important, particularly when exposure occurs by the natural physiological route of inhalation. Differences in target organ dose and toxicity may also be associated with fiber morphology, durability, chemical make-up, and surface properties (Lippmann 1990; Bunn et al. 1991). There is a clear need for experimental systems that provide additional insight into the biological mechanisms and those fiber characteristics that are their determinants. The objective of this paper is to review the experimental literature on the toxicity and carcinogenicity of man-made vitreous fibers (MMVFs) and some other man-made inorganic and organic fibers. The primary focus of this paper is on the use of animal inhalation studies, since these have the greatest utility for risk assessment. A brief discussion is also provided on some possible mechanisms by which fibers induce toxic effects.

MMVFs is a generic expression for fibrous inorganic substances made primarily from raw materials, such as rock, clay, slag, or glass, because of their synthetic, amorphous, glassy nature. MMVFs are also referred to as man-made mineral fibers (MMMFs), but MMVF is preferred because it is more technically correct. These products share a common manufacturing origin in that they are all created from molten masses of raw material under highly controlled conditions. The initial development of some of these fibers occurred in the late 1800s, with development of other fiber types occurring in the 1930s and beyond. Other inorganic and organic man-made fibers that will be covered are potassium titanate (PKT) and potassium octatitanate fibers (Fibex[R]), silicon carbide fibers, carbon fibers, and para-aramid fibers. The development of these fibers has occurred during the past few decades.

RESULTS FROM NONINHALATION STUDIES

Only studies using intraperitoneal or intrapleural injection of man-made fibers (IARC 1988; USEPA 1988) consistently produce serosal cancer. In contrast, the results are equivocal for intratracheal instillation. Positive intratracheal studies using fibrous glass have been reported only by Pott and colleagues (Mohr et al. 1984; Pott et al. 1987), whereas negative studies have been reported by Gross (1976), Wright and Kuschner (1977), Feron et al. (1985), and Smith et al. (1987).

Although there is some dissenting opinion, the consensus of the experts in the field is that the weaknesses of noninhalation studies of fibrous materials severely limit their relevance for human risk assessment (IPCS 1988; USEPA 1988; NIEHS 1989). The limitations include the following:

1. Excessive or overload doses.
2. Normal respiratory defense mechanisms are bypassed.
3. Little or no chance for natural clearance of fiber from the injection site.
4. Abnormal anatomical localization of fibers.
5. Little opportunity for dissolution or fragmentation in body tissues.
6. Little or no interaction with cell types common in the terminal bronchioles and alveoli.

Studies from noninhalation in vivo routes of administration may also be of questionable relevance because the rate and extent at which fibers reach target tissues are much greater than what could possibly occur after inhalation exposure. Thus, pathogenesis from intratracheal, intraperitoneal, or intrapleural administration of fibers may simply be a consequence of "overload" doses to locations that, under a physiological exposure scenario, may never occur (NIEHS 1989).

When fibers are administered via intracavity injections, the anatomic fate and potential for normal clearance, leaching, degradation, fragmentation, or any other transformations are not necessarily the same as after inhalation. Some of these transformations are known to influence pathogenesis. Thus, fibers injected into target tissue areas may be qualitatively and quantitatively different compared with fibers that have been inhaled and translocated to target tissue.

The results of fiber studies using noninhalation in vivo routes of administration may be no more relevant than the results of short-term in vitro screening tests for risk assessment. Noninhalation in vivo studies and short-term in vitro studies have the following similarities: (1) the test agent is placed directly onto target cells; (2) virtually all physiological barriers that normally impede and/or prevent the test agent from reaching the target cells are removed; and (3) the test agent is introduced at a rate and extent much greater than if the test subject were exposed by inhalation, which is the most probable route of human exposure. The primary advantage of the noninhalation in vivo models over in vitro tests is that the long observation period allows for the development of tumors. Noninhalation in vivo models and in vitro tests may have use as screening tests for determining the relative toxicities of fibers or for understanding mechanisms of fiber toxicity but are of no use for risk assessment.

FIBER INHALATION STUDIES

General Considerations

The animal model chosen must be capable of induction of asbestos-related disease observed in humans by inhalation. It is important that studies of chronic diseases be of adequate length for tumors with long latencies to develop. A chronic study should include adequate exposure and total observation periods. For example, in particulate inhalation studies, rats are now usually exposed for 2 years, which is a standard approach for studying all types of materials for chronic toxicity/carcinogenicity studies. Furthermore, animals should be observed for their lifetime or until 20% survival of the test group is observed. It is also important to have positive and sham-exposed negative controls.

Inhalation is the only natural route of exposure for fibers to the target organs in humans. Thus, in designing animal experiments, the techniques of fiber preparation, aerosolization, measuring exposures, and determining actual target organ dose are critical. Special techniques are often necessary to assure adequate target organ dose by inhalation. The fiber used must be of dimensions that permit deposition into the deep lung regions (i.e., respirable fibers) for the model used. For example, in rat models, it is estimated that the majority of fibers that are 1 μm wide x 20 μm long are respirable, and fibers longer than 200 μm will be intercepted in the airways. In addition, nasal rather than whole-body exposure is preferred in fiber-inhalation studies. For example, the quantities of specially sized fibers required for whole-body exposure are prohibitive, and nasal exposure levels are more controllable.

The characteristics of the fiber aerosol in actual work areas for humans is also an important consideration. For example, an average fiber size of 1 μm wide x 20 μm long has been measured using simulated refractory ceramic fibers (RCF) work practices. Therefore, it is critical to use fibers that are preselected for their size and to verify the actual size distributions of the fiber-exposure aerosol. Nonfibrous particles should also be minimized. Furthermore, fiber preparation, handling, and aerosolization must not alter the physical-chemical characteristics of the fiber because, as will be discussed below, these are critical determinants of fiber toxicity (Bunn et al. 1991; Hesterberg et al. 1991a).

To assure quality control, the lofting technique and exposure level should be regularly monitored during the study by both gravimetric and fiber-counting techniques. Finally, lung ashing or other methods of fiber recovery should be performed at selected times during the study to determine total dose levels to the lung.

The number of animals tested must be sufficient to achieve the statistical goals of the study. This aspect of the design of the experiment requires knowledge, such as the background incidence of the disease(s) of interest in the species and the likely attrition of the animal from disease before senescence.

Selection of Exposure Concentrations

Another vital study design consideration is the selection of exposure concentrations. It is important that at least three exposure concentrations be used in the chronic inhalation study in order to determine the dose-response relationship of any changes induced. The highest concentration used should be the "maximum tolerated dose" (MTD), and lower concentrations can be 50% of the MTD and multiples of the projected occupational and environmental exposure levels. MTD is defined as "that dose which, when given for the duration of the chronic study as the highest dose, will not shorten the treated animal's longevity from any toxic effects other than the induction of neoplasms. The MTD should not cause morphologic evidence of toxicity of a severity that would interfere with the interpretation of the study" (NTP 1984; McConnell 1989). In actuality, as applied to carcinogenesis studies, the concept is little different from what one encounters in most other types of toxicity testing, i.e., tests to determine reproductive toxicity, teratology, immunotoxicity, renal toxicity, neural toxicity, and so forth. A basic premise in fiber toxicology is to administer a sufficiently high enough dose to explore whether a given response is possible.

Additional reasons for using the MTD for carcinogen testing in rodents are as follows:

1. To adjust for the varying sensitivity of the model (rodent). Mice and rats may be more resistant (on a dose basis) to the carcinogenic effects of certain agents than humans.
2. To make up for the limited number of animals used in usual rodent bioassays. It is impractical to use thousands of animals, as would be needed to predict the potential effects at lower exposure levels.
3. It is consistent with other approaches in toxicology, as noted above.
4. It provides consistency in design and allows for comparison of the results with other studies.

It has been stated that the major problem with the MTD is not the scientific basis for its use but rather that "we don't like the results we obtain from such studies" (McConnell 1989). It needs to be stressed that the results of a carcinogenesis bioassay conducted at an MTD do not necessarily indicate that the test agent is a carcinogen in humans, especially in terms of the human exposure scenario. Such results are only the first step in risk characterization. For this reason, although it is important that an MTD of the fiber under test be administered, lower concentrations will provide dose-response data that will assist in risk assessment if pathological effects are induced. All of the available data need to be evaluated in a "weight-of-the-evidence" approach to determine the true hazard and risk in humans.

MMVF INHALATION STUDIES

The inhalation studies cited in this discussion are summarized in Table 1. Whenever possible, the exposure levels are given in terms of both mass (mg/m^3) and fiber levels (fibers [f]/cm^3). There are predictably varying levels of nonfibrous material in the various studies. In addition, cited fiber levels may not be comparable, since different methodologies have been employed.

Fibrous Glass

A number of chronic inhalation studies of fibrous glass have been conducted previously (Gross et al. 1976; Lee et al. 1981; McConnell et al. 1984; Wagner et al. 1984; LeBouffant et al. 1987; Muhle et al. 1987; Smith et al. 1987), and under these experimental conditions there was a lack of tumor induction (see Table 1 for details of the protocols and results).

Fibrous glass has been tested by inhalation in guinea pigs (one study), hamsters (two studies), and rats (all of the cited studies). Two important studies for use in human risk assessment of fibrous glass exposure were reported by Wagner et al. (1984) and McConnell et al. (1984). In parallel studies, using the same lot of JM100 fibrous glass, these two groups of researchers demonstrated that inhalation exposure of rats to 10 mg/m^3 of the fibrous glass for 12 months resulted in no significant increase in lung tumors during the lifetime of the animals. As noted by the investigators, exposure to a similar mass concentration of chrysotile asbestos resulted in a significant increase in lung tumors.

Another important inhalation study, which suggests that fibrous glass is not tumorigenic in animals, was reported by Smith et al. (1987). In that study, no tumors were observed in rats or hamsters after inhalation exposure to 3–12 mg/m^3 of several different compositions of fibrous glass. The negative tumor finding with JM100 fibrous glass is especially compel-

TABLE 1 *SUMMARY OF MAN-MADE FIBER CHRONIC INHALATION STUDIES*

Study	Fiber characteristics[1]	Test system	Exposure	Findings	Comments
Fibrous Glass					
Gross (1976)	uncoated/coated glass avg. dia., 0.5 μm avg. length, 10 μm	lifetime study 30 rats and 30 hamsters	2 yr 106–135 mg/m^3	no fibrosis or tumors	poor survival
Lee et al. (1981)	fiberglass avg. dia., 1.2 μm length, <2 μm	24-mo. study 46 male S-D rats 33 albino guinea pigs 34 hamsters	90 days 400 mg/m^3 (700 f/cm^3)	no significant tumor increase	short exposure small no. of animals; short fibers
Wagner et al. (1984)	JM 100 FG avg. dia., 0.3 μm length, 71% <10 μm uncoated and coated FG	lifetime study 28 ea. of male and female Fisher 344 rats	12 mo. 10 mg/m^3 (1436 f/cm^3)	no significant tumor increase	
McConnell et al. (1984)	JM 100 FG	lifetime study male and female Fisher 344 rats	12 mo. 10 mg/m^3 (1436 f/cm^3)	no significant tumor increase	

LeBouffant et al. (1987)	JM 100 FG avg. dia., 0.2 μm length, 94% <5 μm glass wool dia., 68% <1 μm length, 59% >10 μm	24-mo. study 24 ea. of male and female Wistar rats	12 or 24 mo. 5 mg/m³ (332 f/cm³)	no fibrosis or significant tumor increase	low fiber concentration
Muhle et al. 1987	JM 104 FG length, 90% <12.4 μm dia., 50% <0.42 μm	lifetime study 107 female Wistar rats	12 mo. 3 mg/m³ (252 f/cm³)	no significant tumor increase	low fiber concentration; no tumors in asbestos groups
Smith et al. 1987	JM 100 FG avg. dia., 0.45 μm avg. length, 4.7 μm	lifetime study 69 male Syrian hamsters 57 female OM rats	24 mo. 3 mg/m³ (3000 f/cm³)	no fibrosis or tumors	3 tumors in asbestos rats (1 mesothelioma, 2 bronchoalveolar tumors); also studied 3 glass wools of >3 μm dia. with no tumor induction

(Continued on following page.)

TABLE 1 (CONTINUED.)

Study	Fiber characteristics[1]	Test system	Exposure	Findings	Comments
Mineral Wool					
Wagner et al. (1984)	rock wool dia., 58% <1 μm length, 68% >10 μm	lifetime study 28 ea. of male and female Fisher 344 rats	12 mo. 10 mg/m³ (227 f/cm³)	no fibrosis or significant tumor increase	
LeBouffant et al. (1987)	rock wool dia., 22.7% <1 μm length, 60% >10 μm	24-mo. study 24 ea. of male and female Wistar rats	24 mo. 5 mg/m³ (11 f/cm³)	no fibrosis or significant tumor increase	very low fiber concentration
Smith et al. (1987)	slag wool avg. dia., 2.7 μm length, 75% >10 μm	lifetime study 69 male Syrian hamsters 55 female OM rats	24 mo. 10 mg/m³ (200 f/cm³)	no fibrosis or tumors	3 tumors in asbestos rats (1 mesothelioma, 2 broncho-alveolar tumors); slag wool fibers relatively thick
RCFs					
Davis et al. (1984)	RCF dia., 90% <0.3μm length, 90% <3 μm	up to 32 mo. 48 Wistar rats	12 mo. 8.4 mg/m³ (95 f/cm³)	interstitial fibrosis lung tumors in 8 rats (1 adenoma, (3 carcinomas, 4 malignant histiocytomas)	mostly short, thin fibers

Smith et al. (1987)	RCF dia., 86% 2 μm length, 83% >10 μm	lifetime study 70 male Syrian hamsters 55 female OM rats	24 mo. 12 mg/m³ (200 f/cm³)	no fibrosis or tumors in rats; one mesothelioma in hamsters	3 tumors in asbestos rats (1 mesothelioma, 2 broncho-alveolar tumors]; no tumors in asbestos-exposed hamsters

Other Man-made Fibers

Lee et al. (1981)	potassium titanate (PKT) avg. dia., 0.2 μm length, 6% >10 μm	24-mo. study 46 male S-D rats 32 albino guinea pigs, 34 hamsters	90 days 70 mg/m³ (2,900 f/cm³)	no significant tumor increase	short exposure small no. animals; short fibers
	postassium octatitanate (Fybex[R]) avg. dia., 0.2 μm length, 18% >10 μm	24-mo. study 40 male S-D rats/dose; 35 albino guinea pigs/dose; 37 hamsters/dose	90 days doses: 40, 80, and 370 mg/m³ (2,900, 13,500, 41,800 f/cm³)	fibrosis at 2 highest conc.; 3 mesotheliomas in hamsters at 2 highest conc.; 2 adenomas and 2 carcinomas in rats	short exposure small no. animals; short fibers
Lee et al. (1988)	ultrafine Kevlar[R] dia., 90% <1.5 μm length, ~60% >10 μm	24-mo. study 100 rats/sex/dose/group	24 mo. at 0.08, 0.32, and 0.63 mg/m³; 12 mo. at 2.23 mg/m³ (2.5, 25, 100, and 400 f/cm³)	fibrosis at conc. ≥ 0.32 mg/m³; significant increase in carcinomas at 0.63 and 2.23 mg/m³	no positive controls

[1]FG represents fibrous glass.

ling because the small diameter of this fiber would have allowed significant deposition in the deep lung. Additional multiple dose studies of two different compositions of fibrous glass are currently underway at Research and Consulting Company (RCC) in Geneva.

Mineral Wool

There have been three reports of chronic inhalation studies conducted with mineral wool: Wagner et al. (1984), LeBouffant et al. (1987), and Smith et al. (1987) (Table 1). As was seen with fibrous glass, all three studies have shown no tumorigenic response by this route of exposure. The studies by Wagner et al. and LeBouffant et al. were lifetime studies of rats breathing rock wool. No significant increase in tumor incidence was observed in the mineral-wool-exposed animals in either study, whereas 25% and 19% incidences of tumors, respectively, were observed in animals treated with chrysotile asbestos.

Smith et al. (1987) reported that exposing rats and hamsters to 10 mg/m³ of mineral wool (slag wool) for 24 months resulted in no tumors. The incidence of tumors in the control group exposed to short crocidolite asbestos did not statistically increase. Additional dose-response studies of two different compositions of mineral wool have been initiated at RCC in Geneva.

RCFs

There are three known chronic inhalation studies of RCFs. Two investigations have been completed and published (Table 1): one by Davis et al. (1984) and the other by Smith et al. (1987). A third chronic inhalation study, which exposes rats and hamsters to the MTD of RCFs, will be completed in 1990 or early 1991 (Imamura et al. 1990; Bunn et al. 1991; Hesterberg et al. 1991; D.M. Bernstein, pers. comm.).

Davis exposed 48 rats to RCFs by inhalation for 7 hours a day, 5 days a week, over a period of 224 days. The airborne dose of fibers more than 5 μm long was reported to be 95 f/cm³. Animals sacrificed at the end of the study were reported to have an average of 5% pulmonary fibrosis, and eight of the rats were found to have pulmonary tumors with three animals demonstrating lung carcinomas. There was also one peritoneal mesothelioma reported.

Smith et al. (1987) exposed hamsters and rats to RCFs at 200 f/cm³, for 6 hours a day, 5 days a week, for 24 months. The experiments involving rats reported no cancer and little pulmonary fibrosis; this conflicts sharply with the Davis study. Inhalation experiments on hamsters reported one cancer (mesothelioma) in 50 animals, but no fibrosis was observed. Of 157 control animals, 1 developed a spontaneous tumor without exposure to fibers.

In the third study, which is not yet complete, specially sized fibers (~ average dimensions: 1 μm wide x 20 μm long) were used to generate a fiber aerosol that was rat respirable. These dimensions represent only averages; the sized fibers have a distribution of different lengths and diameters. Groups of rats were exposed for 6 hours a day, 5 days a week to the MTD (30 mg/m³, ~200–250 f/cm³) of four different types of RCFs. Hamsters were exposed to only kaolin RCFs. Positive controls (chrysotile asbestos) and negative controls (filtered air) were included in both the rat and the hamster studies.

Interim sacrifices have revealed lung fibrosis beginning at 9 months and the development of malignant mesothelioma in 36 of 102 hamsters (35%) exposed to RCFs (Hesterberg et al. 1991). The rat inhalation study is not yet complete, but levels of lung fibrosis similar to those in the hamster study were observed at interim sacrifices in this species (Hesterberg et al. 1991). An additional chronic inhalation study of multiple concentrations of RCFs in rats has been initiated to provide data for risk assessment of these fibers.

INHALATION STUDIES OF OTHER MAN-MADE FIBERS

PKT and Potassium Octatitanate

Lee et al. (1981) studied the pulmonary responses to chronic inhalation exposure of respirable PKT and potassium octatitanate (Fybex^R) fibers in rats, hamsters, and guinea pigs, and compared them with the effects produced by amosite asbestos (Table 1). PKT induced no significant increase in tumor incidence, whereas Fybex[R] induced three mesotheliomas in hamsters and a number of airway tumors in rats at concentrations of 80 and 370 mg/m^3.

There were marked species differences in the pulmonary responses to these fibers. In general, the degree of lung fibrosis was slightly more marked in hamsters than in guinea pigs but less than in rats. On the other hand, Fibex[R]-exposed hamsters were more susceptible to the development of pleural fibrosis than exposed rats or guinea pigs. Because this study suffers from a number of limitations, such as the use of a small number of animals and a short duration of exposure, definitive assessments of the fibrogenic and carcinogenic potential of Fybex[R] and PKT fibers cannot be made. The results of the study by Lee et al. (1981) also indicate that the hamster may be a more sensitive animal model for the induction of pleural mesothelioma and pleural fibrosis via inhalation than the rat. However, the rat is known to be a sensitive model for pulmonary fibrosis and lung tumors.

Silicon Carbide

Although no chronic inhalation studies have been reported on this fiber, silicon carbide fiber has been tested in a subchronic inhalation study in rats (Chamberlain 1985, 1987). In this study, each of five groups of 50 male and 50 female rats were exposed for 6 hours daily, 5 days a week, for 13 weeks to silicon carbide fibers (4.5 μm wide x 0.2 μm long) at average concentrations of 3.93, 10.7, or 60.5 mg/m^3 (630, 1740, or 7276 f/cm^3), crocidolite asbestos (1.5 μm wide x 0.2 μm long) at 1298 f/cm^3, or only filtered air as negative control. From each group, 25 animals were sacrificed at the end of the exposure period. The remaining animals were observed for an additional 26 weeks.

Histologic examination of silicon-carbide-exposed lungs showed a dose-related increase in the incidence and severity of adenomatous hyperplasia of the lung along with alveolar wall thickening. In addition, there were dose-related pleural changes including subpleural inflammatory lesions, minimalto-mild visceral pleural fibrosis, and visceral and parietal pleural hyperplasia. None of the above pathological changes had subsided in incidence or severity at the end of a 26-week recovery period. In fact, pleural-thickening incidence and adenomatous hyperplasia incidence and severity were found to be increased at that time. Because of the unresolved pathological lesions in the lung after the recovery period and because pleural thickening and adenomatous hyperplasia may progress under some situations to tumor formation, the carcinogenic potential of silicon carbide cannot be ruled out. There was no significant inflammatory or fibrotic activity in the crocidolite group, which was attributed to small fiber length.

The combined results of available experimental studies lend support to recent epidemiologic findings showing respiratory effects associated with the silicon carbide fiber industry (Peters et al. 1984; Smith et al. 1984; Gauthier et al. 1985; Osterman et al. 1989). Chronic rodent inhalation studies using multiple doses of this fiber may be needed to assess more definitively the carcinogenic risk of this fiber to man.

Carbon Fiber

Two short-term and one subchronic inhalation studies were conducted in an attempt to evaluate the pulmonary effects of carbon fibers (Holt and Horne 1978; Holt 1982; Owen et al. 1986). However, all of these studies are considered inadequate because of the extremely low concentration of respirable carbon fibers and the short duration of exposure and observation.

Aramid Fibers

The pathogenic potential of para-aramid fibers was investigated in a chronic inhalation study by Lee et al. (1988). Details of the protocol and results of this study are found in Table 1. Briefly, groups of male and female rats were exposed for 2 years to various concentrations of ultrafine Kevlar[R] fibrils up to 2.33 mg/m^3. A low level of lung fibrosis was seen in exposed rats at the three highest concentrations. In addition, exposed animals showed dose-related lung lesions characterized by alveolar type II cell hyperplasia, bronchoalveolar hyperplasia and bronchiolization, collagen fiber granulomas, and cholesterol-containing granulomas.

A dose-related increase in lung tumors identified as cystic keratinizing squamous cell carcinomas was found in female rats exposed to the two highest dose levels. In addition, 1 of 36 males (3%) of the high-dose group developed lung tumors. One limitation of this study is that it was terminated at 24 months, rather than continuing for the lifetime of the animals (or 20% survival). It is not uncommon for most of the tumors to arise after 24 months in chronic particulate inhalation studies.

MECHANISMS OF ACTION FOR FIBER TOXICITY AND CARCINOGENICITY

The mechanisms whereby inhaled fibers result in pathological changes in the respiratory tract and lining surfaces of the chest and abdominal cavities are not completely understood. Nevertheless, certain principles of biological activity have been elucidated that appear to explain the differing responses to fibers on the basis of size, geometry, durability, and to a lesser extent, chemical composition (Mossman et al. 1983; Lippmann 1988).

Deposition and Clearance

Fiber size and geometry are the determinants of host entry and intrapulmonic distribution. The essential determinant of entry is the aerodynamic diameter (Stober 1972). The aerodynamic diameter of a fiber is approximated by the formula $D_A = 1.3(p^{1/2}d^{5/6}L^{1/6})$, where D_A is the aerodynamic diameter, p is the density, d is the diameter, and L is the fiber length.

Fibers of an aerodynamic diameter greater than 12 μm are not likely to reach the target areas (bronchioles and alveoli) in humans, whereas fibers of an aerodynamic diameter greater than 6 μm are not likely to reach the target areas in rodents (Schlesinger 1987). The ability of the rodent nose to filter out 90–95% of the inhaled fibers accounts for most of this difference. Therefore, although both aspects of size (length and diameter) are important, the diameter of fibers appears to be of greater significance in relation to initial deposition and to their translocation within the lung and their extension to the pleural and peritoneal surfaces. The length of the fiber does have an impact on the ability of the lung to clear the fiber once it reaches the target area, i.e., longer fibers are not cleared as effectively as shorter fibers.

Durability

Although dimension controls the entry and final site of deposition in the lung, durability is the critical basis for the accumulation of a lung burden of fibers. Numerous investigators have shown that in the case of asbestos, the amphibole, the more durable fiber type, accumulates in human lungs in quantities that correlate with cumulative exposure, whereas chrysotile, a less-durable fiber, does not (for review, see Mossman et al. 1990).

Evidence from animal experiments indicates that fibers are attacked by fluids normally present in the lung (Morgan and Holmes 1986; Bellman et al. 1987). This can cause fragmentation to shorter fibers that are biologically less active and are more readily removed from the lungs by clearance mechanisms or can even lead to the total dissolution. It is therefore thought that some man-made fibers may be less toxic and less likely to cause lung tumors in the animals because they are more soluble and do not remain in the lung long enough to cause damage.

The lack of durability of fibers has also been demonstrated in the laboratory using physiological solutions that simulate the natural lung environment. The dissolution rate of mineral fibers has been shown to be dependent on chemical composition and can differ between fiber types by several orders of magnitude (Law et al. 1990). Other factors that may affect the intrapulmonic anatomic fate are the rigidity of fibers, their surface properties, and fiber-end architecture (e.g., smooth, grainy, or spiculed edges) (Lippmann 1988, 1990).

Although asbestos fibers do vary significantly in their neoplasm-producing potential, it is clear that dose, dimension, and durability are crucial, although not exclusive, determinants of oncogenicity. Two sites of oncogenic effect have been verified in the lung and in the pleura surrounding the lung, i.e., bronchogenic carcinoma and mesothelioma (Demy and Adler 1967; McDonald et al. 1974).

Bronchogenic Carcinoma

The primary site of response of the lungs to fiber inhalation is at the level of respiratory bronchioles, alveolar ducts, and alveoli. The initial response to deposition of fiber in the alveoli is an alveolitis with fluid exudation and inflammatory cell infiltration. The fibrogenic process originates in the bronchiolar-alveolar region with fibrosis initially becoming manifest in the peribronchiolar regions.

One potential mechanism of action for the induction of lung cancer is the fibrosis that is the result of the release of endogenous mediators of fibrosis and epithelial proliferation. The theoretical mechanism of development for bronchogenic carcinoma is the replacement of the normal architecture of the peripheral lung parenchyma by scar, leading to anatomic deformity, and epithelial proliferation that provides a milieu similar to that reported in studies of scar cancer in the past. The sequestered or entrapped pulmonary epithelium is more susceptible to malignant transformation and carcinoma development.

A second possible mechanism of action is a direct genotoxic effect, as suggested by cell-culture studies. Several studies have shown that concentrations of asbestos and MMMFs that induce neoplastic transformation of cells in culture also induce mutations at the chromosomal level, including chromosomal aberrations and numerical changes. These findings suggest that mineral fibers may act by a direct genotoxic mechanism to induce neoplasms. (Hesterberg and Barrett 1984; Oshimura et al. 1984; Jaurand et al. 1986).

Mesothelioma

Malignant neoplasms arising from mesothelial surfaces have been described in the pleura, pericardium, and peritoneum with asbestos and erionite. The initial step in the development of malignant mesothelioma is the translocation of fibers to the pleura, peritoneum, or pericardium. The induction of fibrosis has been theorized to be a required antecedent for mesothelioma development much in the manner of the development of malignant neoplasms after the subcutaneous implantation of solid-state materials (e.g., plastics and metal). Solid-state carcinogenesis studies have shown that the pattern of fibrosis with implants is similar to the fibrosis seen in the pleura exposed to fibers. The potential genotoxicity of the fibers deposited in the pleural space is a second potential mechanism of action. Lechner et al. (1985) have shown that chromosomal aberrations are associated with asbestos-induced transformation of human mesothelial cells in culture.

SUMMARY AND CONCLUSIONS

Studies clearly show increased risks of lung cancer, mesothelioma, and nonmalignant respiratory disease associated with the inhalation of naturally occurring mineral fibers. The study of fiber carcinogenesis in animal models for use in human risk assessment requires special techniques to assure adequate physiological dose to the target organs. Inhalation exposure is necessary. Furthermore, fiber preparation, aerosolization, measuring exposures, and determining actual target organ dose are critical. Noninhalation in vivo models and in vitro tests may have use as screening tests for determining the relative toxicities of fibers or for understanding mechanisms of fiber toxicity but are of no use for risk assessment.

A number of chronic inhalation studies have been conducted using man-made fibers. The results vary, depending on protocol and fiber type. Several studies using MMVFs are in progress. It is anticipated that the results of these studies will further the understanding of the determinants of fiber carcinogenesis.

Several known and theoretical determinants of fiber tumorigenicity are (1) the ability to gain entry into the lung, (2) translocation within and out of the lung, (3) clearance from the respiratory tract, (4) durability in body fluids, (5) induction of cellular components of the acute inflammatory response, (6) the initiation of fibrosis and cell proliferation, and (7) induction of direct genotoxic changes. The foregoing are in turn critically related to the dose (concentration x time at the target tissue), fiber size, geometry, surface area and charge, and possible cofactor effects of exposure to toxic inhalants or the presence of antecedent or concurrent disease.

ACKNOWLEDGMENT

The opinions expressed in this article do not necessarily reflect the official position or policies of the United States Environmental Protection Agency.

REFERENCES

Bellmann, B., H. Muhle, F. Pott, H. Konig, H. Kloppel, and K. Spurny. 1987. Persistence of man-made mineral fibres (MMMF) and asbestos in rat lungs. *Ann. Occup. Hyg.* **31:** 693.

Bunn, W.B., T.W. Hesterberg, G. Chase, and R. Anderson. 1991. Manmade mineral fibers. In *Medical toxicology of hazardous materials.* Williams and Wilkins, Baltimore, Maryland. (In press.)

Chamberlain, W.T. 1985, 1987. *Subchronic (39 week) inhalation toxicity study of silicon carbide fibers in rats.* U.S. Environmental Protection Agency File no. 8EHQ-0287-0574, Washington, D.C.

Davis, J.M.G., J. Addison, R.E. Bolton, K. Donaldson, A.D. Jones, and A. Wright. 1984. The pathogenic effects of fibrous ceramic aluminum silicate glass administered to rats by inhalation or peritoneal injection. In *Biological effects of man-made mineral fibres. Proceedings of a WHO/IARC Conference,* vol. 2, p. 303. World Health Organization, Copenhagen.

Demy, N.G. and H. Adler. 1967. Asbestos and malignancy. *Am. J. Roentgenol.* **100:** 597.

Feron, V.J., P.M. Scherrenberg, H.R. Immel, and B.J. Spit. 1985. Pulmonary response of hamsters to glasswool fiber: Chronic effects of repeated intratracheal instillation with or without benzo[a]pyrene. *Carcinogenesis* **6:** 1495.

Gauthier, J.J., H. Ghezzo, and R.R. Martin. 1985. Pneumoniosis following carborundum (silicon carbide) exposure. *Am. Rev. Respir. Dis.* **131:** 191.

Gross, P. 1976. The effects of glasswool fiber dust on the lung of animals. In *Occupational exposure to glasswool fiber. HEW Publ. no.* **76-151:** 166.

Hesterberg, T.W. and J.C. Barrett. 1984. Dependence of asbestos and mineral dust-induced transformation of mammalian cells in culture upon fiber dimension. *Cancer Res.* **44:** 2170.

Hesterberg, T.W., R. Mast, E.E. McConnell, J. Chevalier, D.M. Bernstein, W.B. Bunn, and R. Anderson. 1991a. Chronic inhalation toxicity of refractory ceramic fibers in Syrian hamsters. *NATO ASI Ser. Ser. A Life Sci.* (in press).

Hesterberg, T.W., R. Mast, E.E. McConnell, O. Vogel, J. Chevalier, D.M. Bernstein, and R. Anderson. 1991b. Chronic inhalation toxicity and oncogenicity study of refractory ceramic fibers in Fisher 344 rats. *Toxicologist* **11**: 85.

Holt, P.F. 1982. Submicron carbon dust in the guinea pig. *Environ. Res.* **28**: 434.

Holt, P.F. and M. Horne. 1978. Dust from carbon fibre. *Environ. Res.* **17**: 276.

Imamura, T., O. Vogel, J. Chevalier, R. Mast, T.W. Hesterberg, R. Anderson, and D. Bernstein. 1990. Evaluation of pulmonary functions during chronic inhalation studies with refractory ceramic fibers (RCF) and an experimental fiber in rats. *Toxicologist* **10**: 7.

International Agency for Research on Cancer (IARC). 1988. Man-made mineral fibres and radon. In *IARC monographs on the evaluation of carcinogenic risks to humans*, vol. 43. Lyon, France.

International Programme on Chemical Safety (IPCS). 1988. *Man-made mineral fibres.* Environmental Health Criteria 77. World Health Organization, Geneva, Switzerland.

Jaurand, M.C., L. Kheuand, L. Magne, and J. Bignon. 1986. Chromosomal changes induced by chrysotile fibres or benzo(3-4)pyrene in rat pleural mesothelial cells. *Mutat. Res.* **169**: 141.

Law, B., W.B. Bunn, and T.W. Hesterberg. 1990. Solubility of polymeric organic fibers and man-made vitreous fibers in gambles solution. *Inhalation Toxicol.* **2**: 321.

LeBouffant, L., H. Daniel, J.P. Henin, J.C. Martin, C. Normand, G. Thichoux, and F. Trolard. 1987. Experimental study on long-term effects of inhaled MMMF on the lung of rats. *Ann. Occup. Hyg.* **31**: 765.

Lechner, J.F., T. Tokiwa, M. La Veck, W.F. Benedict, S. Banks-Schlegel, H. Yeager, Jr., A. Banerjee, and C.C. Harris. 1985. Asbestos-associated chromosomal changes in human mesothelial cells. *Proc. Natl. Acad. Sci.* **82**: 3884.

Lee, K.P., C.E. Barras, F.D. Griffith, R.S. Waritz, and C.A. Lapin. 1981. Comparative pulmonary responses to inhaled inorganic fibers with asbestos and fiberglass. *Environ. Res.* **24**: 167.

Lee, K.P, O.P. Kelly, O. O'Neal, J.C. Stadler, and G.L. Kennedy, Jr. 1988. Lung response to ultrafine Kevlar aramid synthetic fibrils following 2-year inhalation exposure in rats. *Fundam. Appl. Toxicol.* **11**: 1.

Lippmann, M. 1988. Review: Asbestos exposure indices. *Environ. Res.* **46**: 86.

———. 1990. Man-made mineral fibers (MMMF): Human exposures and health risk assessment. *Toxicol. Ind. Health* **6**: 225.

McConnell, E.E. 1989. The maximum tolerated dose: The debate. *J. Am. Coll. Toxicol.* **8**: 1115.

McConnell, E.E., J.C. Wagner, J.W. Skidmore, and J.A. Moore. 1984. A comparative study of the fibrogenic and carcinogenic effects of UICC Canadian chrysotile B asbestos and glass microfibre (JM 100). In *Biological effects of man-made mineral fibres. Proceedings of a WHO/IARC Conference*, vol. 2, p. 234. World Health Organization, Copenhagen.

McDonald, J.C., M.R. Becklake, G.W. Gibbs, A.D. McDonald, and D.E. Rossiter. 1974. The health of chrysotile asbestos mine and mill workers of Quebec. *Arch. Environ. Health* **38:** 61.

Mohr, U., F. Pott, and F.J. Vonnahmo. 1984. Morphological aspects of mesotheliomas after intratracheal instillation of fibrous dusts in Syrian golden hamsters. *Exp. Pathol.* **26:** 179.

Morgan, A. and A. Holmes. 1986. Solubility of asbestos and man-made mineral fibers in vitro and in vivo: Its significance in lung disease. *Environ. Res.* **39:** 475.

Mossman, B.T., W.G. Light, and E.Y. Wei. 1983. Asbestos: Mechanisms of toxicity and carcinogenicity in the respiratory tract. *Annu. Rev. Pharmacol. Toxicol.* **23:** 595.

Mossman, B.T., J. Bignon, M. Corn, A. Seaton, and J.B.L. Gee. 1990. Asbestos: Scientific developments and implications for public policy. *Science* **247:** 294.

Muhle, H., F. Pott, B. Bellmann, S. Takenaka, and U. Ziem. 1987. Inhalation and injection experiments in rats to test the carcinogenicity of MMMF. *Ann. Occup. Hyg.* **31:**755.

National Institute of Environmental Health Sciences (NIEHS). 1989. *NIEHS workshop on fibre toxicology research needs.* Research Triangle Park, North Carolina.

National Toxicology Program (NTP). 1984. *Report of the NTP ad hoc panel on chemical carcinogenesis testing and evaluation.* Research Triangle Park, North Carolina.

Oshimura, M., T.W. Hesterberg, T. Tsutsui, and J.C. Barrett. 1984. Correlation of asbestos-induced cytogenetic effects with cell transformation of Syrian hamster embryo cells in culture. *Cancer Res.* **44:** 5017.

Osterman, I.A. Greaves, T.J. Smith, S.K. Hammon, J.M. Robins, and G. Theriault. 1989. Work related decrement in pulmonary function in silicon carbide production workers. *Br. J. Ind. Med.* **46:** 708.

Owen, P., J.R. Glaister, B. Ballantyne, and J.J. Clary. 1986. Subchronic inhalation toxicology of carbon fibers. *J. Occup. Med.* **28:** 373.

Peters, J.M., T.J. Smith, W.E. Belstein Wright, and S.K. Hammond. 1984. Pulmonary effects of exposures in silicon carbide manufacturing. *Br. J. Ind. Med.* **41:** 109.

Pott, F., H.W. Schlipköter, U. Ziem, K. Spurny, and F. Huth. 1987. Carcinogenicity studies on fibres, metal compounds, and some other dusts in rats. *Exp. Pathol.* **32:** 129.

Schlesinger, R.B. 1987. Comparative deposition of inhaled aerosols in experimental animals and humans: A review. *J. Tox. Environ. Health* **15:** 197.

Smith, T.J., S.K. Hammond, F. Laidlaw, and S. Fine. 1984. Respiratory exposures associated with silicon carbide production: Estimation of cumulative exposures for an epidemiologic study. *Br. J. Ind. Med.* **41:** 100.

Smith, D.M., L.W. Ortiz, R.F. Archuleta, and N.F. Johnson. 1987. Long-term health effects in hamsters and rats exposed chronically to man-made vitreous fibers. *Ann. Occup. Hyg.* **31:** 731.

Stanton, M.F. and C. Wrench. 1972. Mechanisms of mesothelioma induction with asbestos and fibrous glass. *J. Natl. Cancer Inst.* **48:** 797.

Stanton, M.F., M. Layard, A. Tegeris, E. Miller, M. May, and E. Kent. 1977. Carcinogenicity of fibrous glass: Pleural response in the rat in relation to fiber dimension. *J. Natl. Cancer Inst.* **58:** 587.

Stanton, M.F., M. Layard, A. Tegeris, E. Miller, M. May, E. Morgan and A. Smith. 1981. Relation of particle dimension to carcinogenicity in amphibole asbestos and other fibrous minerals. *J. Natl. Cancer Inst.* **67:** 965.

Stober, W. 1972. Dynamic shape factors of nonspherical aerosol particles. In *Assessment of airborne particles* (ed. T.T. Mercer et al.), p. 249. Charles C. Thomas, Springfield, Illinois.

U.S. Environmental Protection Agency (USEPA). 1988. *Health hazard assessment of nonasbestos fibers.* Health and Environmental Review Division, Office of Toxic Substances, Washington, D.C.

Wagner, J.C., G.B. Berry, R.J. Hill, D.E. Munday, and J.W. Skidmore. 1984. Animal experiments with MMM(V)F—Effects of inhalation and intrapleural inoculation in rats. In *Biological effects of man-made mineral fibres. Proceedings of a WHO/IARC Conference,* vol. 2, p. 209. World Health Organization, Copenhagen.

Wright, G.W. and M. Kuschner. 1977. The influence of varying lengths of glass and asbestos fibres on tissue response in guinea pigs. In *Inhaled particles IV,* part 1 (ed. W.H. Walton), p. 455. Pergammon Press, Oxford, England.

Index